Quit

Miriam

Miriam Stoppard, MD MRCP practised clinical medicine
for seven years specialising in dermatology for the last
three before joining a major drug company working in
clinical research.

She was Medical Director, then Managing Director
before leaving in 1980 to devote herself full-time to
writing and broadcasting and medical education. She
was Radio London's resident phone-in doctor from
1970–1972 and appeared in *Kaleidoscope, Woman's Hour*
and *Tuesday Call.* Dr Stoppard was medical presenter
on television's *Don't Ask Me, Don't Just Sit There, The
Health Show, Where There's Life* and the BBC TV series *So
You Want to Stop Smoking.*

Dr Stoppard has written on medical matters for 'New
Scientist', 'Vogue', 'Cosmopolitan', 'Homes and Gar-
dens' and is a regular contributor to 'Family Circle'.
She is the author of *Miriam Stoppard's Book of Babycare,
Miriam Stoppard's Book of Health Care, Your Baby* and
Every Woman's Lifeguide.

Dr Stoppard is married to the playwright Tom Stoppard and has two sons and two stepsons.

QUIT SMOKING

MIRIAM STOPPARD

ARIEL BOOKS
BRITISH BROADCASTING CORPORATION

Acknowledgement is due to the following for their kind permission to reprint information:

DR M. A. H. RUSSELL and THE PRACTITIONER for the chart on page 94;

THE LANCET for the charts on pages 49 and 73;

THE ROYAL COLLEGE OF PHYSICIANS for the charts on pages 26, 30, 31, 51, 70, 72, 74 and 75, from *The Third Report of the Royal College of Physicians* 'Smoking *OR* Health' published by Pitman Medical & Scientific;

SIR RICHARD DOLL, CBE and The Editor of the British Medical Journal for the charts on page 50, from The British Medical Association Journal 1976, 4, 1525.

Diagrams by Hugh Ribbans

© Miriam Stoppard 1982
First published 1982

Published by the British Broadcasting Corporation
35 Marylebone High Street, London W1M 4AA

Typeset by Phoenix Photosetting, Chatham,
Printed in Great Britain by Mackays of Chatham Ltd

ISBN 0 563 16541 3

Contents

Acknowledgements

I should like to thank Anna Jackson, the producer of the BBC television series *So You Want To Stop Smoking*, for her help and enthusiasm which continued long after the cameras had stopped rolling. The mountains of research papers on smoking which she put at my disposal made the job of writing a book on stopping smoking a great deal easier and faster than it would otherwise have been. I am grateful to my friend and colleague, Dr John Farquhar of Stanford University, California, for allowing me to refer to the work of the Stanford Heart Disease Prevention Programme on stress management, stress control and smoking cessation contained in his book *The American Way of Life Need Not Be Harmful to Your Health*.
My thanks also to David Simpson of ASH for reading the text and making many helpful comments.

Miriam Stoppard

1 How this book can help you

The major supposition of this book is that you want to give up smoking. It is not going to encourage you to take half measures. It won't suggest that you can be satisfied with cutting down, changing to cigars or starting to smoke a pipe. It is tough and unequivocal. It asks you to give up tobacco of all kinds for the rest of your life.

What it asks is much easier for some than they ever expected. However the majority of people think that it is going to be difficult and this is an obstacle. You may have tried to give up smoking before and, having failed, may feel disheartened. You may not want to try again. A few of you really will find it difficult.

What this book will make you realise is this: if you want to give up smoking, there is nothing that can stop you. Even though you think you don't have enough will-power, you will find it. This book can't help you to want to give up smoking but, if you want to, it can help you not only to stop but, more important, to stay stopped.

Having been a smoker myself, I am only too well aware of all these difficulties and I have tried to structure the book to give you the best possible help in a simple, clear and practical way.

You will still have to make quite an effort regardless of what you have been told or read, there is no substitute for will-power, and it is only by using your will-power that you will become a non-smoker. Don't doubt for one minute that you lack the will-power. You certainly don't. I hope that through and with this book, you will find that you have more will-power than you ever thought, and be proud of it. More than eight million people in Great Britain have stopped smoking. They found the will-power. You can join them.

This book will give you step-by-step guide lines – a blue-print – a programme to help you to stop smoking. It sets out to answer most of the questions you have ever had about giving up smoking. It won't hesitate to give you firm advice and point you in the right direction. It aims to give you support – support when your will-power may flag, when the craving gets great, when you feel like giving up, even if your guard slips and you take a cigarette. It will cheer you up, prop you up, and keep you going. It is a friend. The book is tailor-made for your needs and is prepared for how you may feel at any time while you are giving up. There is something in it somewhere that will help you over the sticky patches.

Keep it with you. Put it in your pocket or your handbag. Turn to it if you need to refresh your memory about some of the things you should be doing. Dip into it when the going gets tough. Re-read its messages, so that you believe them and you think positively. It is the kind of friend that you can refer to at any time, and be sure that you will get suggestions on how to cope with difficult situations. Like the best sort of friend it will boost your morale. Because it is such a supportive friend, don't go anywhere without it, then you can refer to it wherever you are. This book is alive. It will go through your stopping smoking with you – make it your constant companion.

Trust it, rely on it, it will help to help you to stop smoking and that's a promise.

This is a good news book. There is lots of good news about stopping smoking. Stopping in itself is good news. You are joining the non-smokers, and they are healthier, better off, and more attractive than you because they have stopped. You may not have realised that.

1 Stopping can be much easier than you think. Very few people experience the horror stories about unconquerable cravings, impossible bad temper, and excessive weight gain. Once they have stopped, a lot of non-smokers say if they'd known it was going to be so easy, they would have done it years ago.

2 People are more successful at giving up smoking than you may think. After all, nearly nine million people in Great Britain managed to give up smoking and so can you.

3 The craving for cigarettes usually lasts no more than a few weeks at the most, so the worst is over in a relatively short time. The craving for *each* cigarette lasts no more than a few minutes at the most, so you can get around that with fairly simple distractions, eg chewing gum, an apple, drinking a glass of water or taking a walk.

4 You are much more resourceful than you think. If you are creative and determined (and the book gives you quite a lot of

useful tips on how to draw up a cessation programme that is particularly suited to you) you will be able to think up ways of doing without the most difficult cigarettes of the day.

5 You are stronger than you think. No-one is proud of being ruled by smoking, and there is no need to be. You can conquer it.

6 You don't have to put on weight either, (see Chapter 3) but if you find yourself nibbling there will be advice on how to nibble at the right things.

7 The benefits of stopping are almost the best part; better health, more money, no smell, greater enjoyment of food – the list goes on and on.

I *envy* smokers. The minute you give up smoking, you enter lower risk groups for death from a heart attack, bronchitis, emphysema and cancer of the lung. There is no other single step that is likely to improve your chances of health so significantly so quickly.

As of now, you are starting on a programme to stop smoking. This programme covers about five weeks, and goes in steps. There are ten chapters in the book and I would suggest that you read two chapters a week, or alternatively that you at least concentrate on two chapters a week. It doesn't have to be a week, it could be a few days. Go at your own speed, proceeding to the next step when you're ready. The reason for suggesting this is that the book is going to ask you to change your attitudes, your habits and your behaviour. You will stand a better chance of being successful if you make sure that you have mastered one step before you go on to the next.

People give up smoking in all sorts of ways, and no doubt you will find a way that is special to you and suits you best. Within your own framework I would like you to consider the results of research about the best way to give up smoking. Nearly all experts on smoking cessation agree that you improve your chances if you stop smoking in steps. We go through these steps in detail further on in the book with the practical help you'll need.

Step 1 THINK about stopping smoking. Think about why *you* want to stop smoking. I am going to ask you to do that this week.

Step 2 DECIDE to stop smoking. This is probably the single most important thing that you do, because it's the source of your will-power.

Step 3 PREPARE yourself for stopping. The importance of good preparation can't be over emphasised. This greatly increases your chance of success.

Step 4 STOP smoking. 'D' Day. Set a date in the very near future and stick to it. Choose the day carefully. Make it special. Make it different from other days.

Step 5 STAY STOPPED. This is the second most important thing you do and possibly the hardest, your aim is to be a non-smoker for the rest of your life. The first few weeks are the hardest. When you get to this step you've really beaten it. Nothing else you do afterwards will be as difficult as what you've already accomplished.

The programme in this book takes each of these steps one at a time, so you have every opportunity to think about and prepare for the next step. During each of the weeks you won't only be thinking about what you are going to do next. There will be information to digest, and there will be a programme of things that you have to do. So be ready for action.

What you have to do this week

Thinking about stopping

If you want to give up smoking, you are in good company. Six out of every ten smokers wish that they could stop. Over the next few days think of *reasons* why you would like to stop. For instance, are there any of your smoking habits which you don't like? It may be nicotine-stained fingers, or the smell of cigarette smoke on your clothes and hair. It just could be the sight of a full ash tray, or the smell of cigarette smoke in the air when you come into a room. It could be your early morning cough or getting out of breath when you run for a bus or run upstairs. It could be the expense, or self-disgust at being hooked on cigarettes. Instead of simply concentrating on the enjoyment you get from smoking, think about the unpleasant aspects of each cigarette, about the things which upset you or frighten you. Make a list of your reasons, and keep it by you. Go over in your mind some of the reasons why *you* would like to stop smoking. Here are some points to think about:

1 With the price at £1 a pack and rising, it is possibly a habit that you can no longer afford. Think what you would do with the money you could save. Think about *how* you would save it, *where* you would save it, the first things that you would spend your savings on.

2 Your smoking is anti-social. The people you spend the best part of your day with may object to you smoking. You may be the only smoker in the office or work group. Your partner may not smoke or may be quite eager to give up smoking with you.

3 More and more children object to their parents smoking, and make no bones about complaining that the car smells, or the smoke hurts their eyes. Even if your children don't voice their complaints, you may want to set them a good example. You may want to give your children a clean environment to grow up in. It is well known that children of smokers are more likely to take up the habit than children whose parents don't smoke, and your children will doubtless be very proud of you if you kick the habit. One of my own greatest rewards when I stopped smoking was the pride my children took in my achievement. The struggle seemed worthwhile when I heard one of my sons saying to a friend 'Oh no, my mum doesn't smoke any more. She's given it up'.

4 If you are never free of a cough or are getting breathless, or find that head colds always go into your chest, concern about your health could be a strong reason for stopping smoking. Make a list of all your reasons. Keep it handy.

Think of *how long* you have been smoking. How many cigarettes do you smoke a day? On average how many puffs do you take out of each cigarette? Someone who smokes twenty cigarettes a day, takes about 78,000 puffs per year. It is easy for you to calculate how many puffs you take a year and therefore how many you have taken in your life. With each puff, you are taking tars, poisons and irritants into your lungs. Have you ever rubbed at a window or tried to clean the walls of a room where someone smokes? Both are covered with a brown sticky deposit from cigarette smoke. Your lungs are covered with a film of exactly the same unpleasant material. When you stop smoking you will be less prone to coughs, sore throats, colds, sinusitis bronchitis, breathlessness and other chest complaints. Here's an easy to refer to list of some of the benefits of giving up smoking. Re-read it any time you want to refresh your memory or increase your resolve to kick the habit. Make your own list too and keep it with you.

1 You will reduce the risk of heart disease, peptic ulcer, bronchitis, emphesyma and lung cancer.

2 You will save money.

3 Food will taste better.

4 You will get rid of the signs of smoking from the house, like dirty messy ash trays, and from yourself, like nicotine-stained fingers and teeth, smelly hair and clothes.

5 You will be fitter in every day life, and join activities with your children and play sports.

6 You will have a healthier baby.

7 You will set a good example to your children.

8 You will have more self respect.

9 You will be a non-smoker and be proud of saying 'No thanks, I don't smoke'.

The majority of people think they know their smoking habits very well, but most of them really don't. People nearly always *underestimate* the number of cigarettes they smoke and *overestimate* how much they need each one. This week you should try to get some idea of *why*, *when* and *how much* you smoke. You'll get some surprises. One of the things that you should do during the first week is to record on a chart every cigarette you smoke.

For each cigarette you smoke you should note down when you want it, why you want it, and how much you want it. Before the first day is over you will have new insight into your smoking habits. The first shock is how *few* cigarettes you really crave. Most cigarettes are simply habit, associated with situations and circumstances. It is very important for you to note these things down because knowledge about yourself is going to make all the difference when you come to give up. At the end of two or three days, you will find a pattern emerging.

No matter how many cigarettes you smoke, you will know in a fairly short time that the majority of cigarettes in a day are going to be quite easy to give up but there may be six or seven that you really want to smoke, and these ones can be difficult. These are at the classic moments when smokers reach for a cigarette – the first cigarette of the day on getting up or with the early morning cup of coffee or tea; the cigarette at coffee break during the morning; the cigarette when you get anxious or stressed; the one you light up when the phone rings; the one when the stress or anxiety is over, to relax; the cigarette with the first evening drink; the cigarette after a meal.

In keeping this chart, you will get a lot of information about yourself and the way you live, and your reasons for smoking. All of these things are important because they are going to tell you how to deal with your habit when you give it up. They are going to help you to plan and prepare. You are going to be aware long before you stop smoking which cigarettes you can *avoid* and which cigarettes you simply have to *face and fight*. You are going to know well ahead of time the situations where temptation will be greatest, and where the most will-power is needed. This book will tell you how to cope with both of these situations.

Recording your smoking pattern will give you quite a lot of insight into yourself and your habits, and why you do things. If stress makes you smoke you are going to have to learn to cope with stress without the cigarettes – problems aren't going to go away because you have a cigarette. Much more important you are going to learn how to overcome stress by controlling it – then you'll need cigarettes less (see page 59).

If cigarettes help you to relax, then a good way to prepare for giving up would be to learn a relaxation technique that works for you, so that the cigarette becomes redundant (see page 62). By the end of a week you are going to know precisely which cigarettes and which situations are going to be a strain. This will give you the opportunity to draw up a very practical plan of how to cope with the problem cigarettes. Because of this you will be less likely to succumb to temptation, and you will gain more strength from each cigarette you don't smoke.

If your resolve to stop smoking weakens during the first week, when you are thinking about it, here are some of the things that you can do to bolster your determination:

1 Think of the people that you know or may have heard of including famous people who died of lung cancer or other smoking-related diseases.

2 Think about the things you don't like about smoking – re-read your list.

3 Think about the reasons why you want to give up smoking – re-read your list.

4 Think of the benefits of stopping smoking – re-read your list.

5 Talk to as many people who have given up smoking as you can – not one of them will have regretted it.

6 Read Chapters 1 and 2 again.

7 Think of the self respect you will gain.

8 Think how much more pleasant you will make life for others.

9 Think of the nearly nine million people in the British Isles who have given up.

10 Think of the money that the tobacco firms spend on persuading you to go on smoking – and how it has worked so far.

11 Keep on saying to yourself over and over again that in five weeks time you will be a non-smoker.

2 Hard facts I

Non-smokers find it hard to understand why smoking can be so pleasurable. All they can see is a dirty, smelly, unhealthy, expensive habit, which not only affects the smoker but makes life uncomfortable for non-smokers.

I understand the pleasures of smoking completely. As an ex-smoker, I lived through all the pleasurable moments that go with smoking. It is worth re-capping. If you understand why you find smoking so pleasurable you will have important information which will help you to cope with difficult moments when you rely on smoking to get you through.

For most people smoking is a habit rather than an addiction. It is a ritual. It is a collection of thoughts, sensations, movements, actions, which all come together and centre on the lighting and smoking of a cigarette. The ritual may be fast or slow. In moments of stress you go through it very quickly. When you are in a more relaxed mood you savour each moment.

The ritual usually starts by thinking about a cigarette. You then reach for or look for the pack or cigarette box. Having found the pack, you cradle it in your hand. It is smooth and attractive. It fits neatly into your palm. You curl your fingers around it. You smooth its surface. You look for your lighter. It may be very beautiful. It may be cleverly designed and crafted. It may have a fascinating pattern on its surface. It may be expensively enamelled. Its action may be very smooth and precisely engineered. Or it can be a disposable throw-away lighter that fits neatly and smoothly between your fingers, with a rough grating action before it bursts into flame. Lighters are playthings, pleasant to finger, grasp, squeeze and rub. So now you have your pack and your lighter, and lighting up is imminent. You can have a cigarette if you want to, or you can wait for a few seconds, but it is a moment to savour.

All this may sound crazy to a non-smoker, but most smokers would say it is so pleasant that they think non-smokers are missing out on something. One of the nicest moments of all is taking the cigarette out of the pack and feeling it long and smooth and round between your fingers. Then there is the enjoyable moment when you put the cigarette between your lips, flick the lighter into flame and light the cigarette. The first time you inhale the smoke is cool and you draw it deep into your lungs. After a second or two with a deep sigh, you let out all the smoke, and as you do so your body either gets ready for action if what you are facing is stress or relaxes and loses its tension if it is the evening and you are sipping your first drink. You play with the cigarette between your fingers. You watch the smoke in a curling thin column spiralling upwards. You involuntarily put the cigarette back into your mouth and suck on it again.

Of course there is more to a cigarette than these aesthetic pleasures. There are the pharmacological ones too. A cigarette 'hits' you very quickly, more quickly than any other drug you can take by mouth, or smoke for that matter. It acts more quickly than marihuana, which usually takes as long as alcohol – 15 to 20 minutes. No, the smoker who wants the effects of nicotine, knows that from the first puff they are no more than about five seconds away. This is what happens:

1 You inhale the cigarette smoke into your mouth, down through your main bronchial tubes and into the lungs.

2 The instant smoke comes up against the moist glistening lining of your mouth and your airways, the nicotine is instantaneously absorbed into the blood stream and starts coursing through your blood vessels to your brain and around your body.

3 The nicotine begins to affect the brain. Even though I had smoked for years, the first puff of the day, in the morning, always made me feel giddy, and that was the direct effect of nicotine on my brain. For most people nicotine has a stimulating effect on the brain, and makes them feel more alert and wakeful.

4 The heart quickly responds to the effect of nicotine by increasing the rate at which it beats and circulates more blood per minute round the body. This ensures a faster supply of oxygen to all your organs and can help if you want to be more active and alert.

5 The walls of blood vessels are stimulated to contract by nicotine. They narrow down and this raises the blood pressure. The effect of nicotine on the heart is antagonistic to the effect of the

drug on arteries. At one and the same time, nicotine makes the heart pump faster, but gives it a greater resistance (a higher blood pressure) against which to pump. The heart is therefore under strain.

6 Nicotine affects the blood by making the platelets stickier and the blood more likely to clot.

7 Certain nerves in the body are stimulated by nicotine, so you may find that you want to go to the lavatory both to empty your bladder, and to move your bowels shortly after having a cigarette.

8 Nicotine reduces tension in the muscles and allows them to relax. This is one of the reasons why smoking seems to relieve stress and helps you to relax.

9 Nicotine can have a calming effect on people who are anxious and worried. This is why it can bring a feeling of tranquility, and help people to cope with stress.

10 Nicotine can stimulate and arouse some people. It can stave off boredom and fatigue and for a short time it can improve concentration.

There isn't an organ in the body which is left unaffected by the nicotine you inhale from a cigarette. Tobacco contains from 1 to 3 per cent of nicotine, a powerful drug which will stimulate or tranquilise you. In small quantities it does both of these things but in larger quantities, the effects are harmful. For instance, small quantities of nicotine will stimulate certain types of nerves, but larger quantities will paralyse them. Nicotine is one of the most powerful poisons known. It is extremely efficient at killing insects, and is widely used as an insecticide. There is enough nicotine in only one small cigarette to kill a grown man, if it is injected into the blood stream.

Pure nicotine is an oily colourless liquid, but when tobacco is burnt, tiny droplets of nicotine are inhaled as part of the smoke. On average you absorb about 2 milligrams of nicotine from each cigarette.

Depending on how it is cured, tobacco will produce nicotine with a fast or slow effect. Cigar and pipe tobacco and some tobaccos which are used to make continental cigarettes are dried in air and have a low sugar content. When this tobacco is burned the smoke is alkaline. Because saliva is alkaline too, nicotine is absorbed from smoke in the mouth very quickly and has a rapid effect. On the other hand British and American tobaccos are cured in artificial heat, which preserves the sugar in the leaf. When the tobacco is burned the smoke is acid. Nicotine is not usually absorbed from this acid smoke until it reaches the lungs and therefore has a comparatively slow effect.

But you are far too clever to be beaten by fast and slow acting cigarettes. Being a habitual smoker, you can adjust your smoking, so that you get the amount of nicotine you like as fast as you want it. Experiments have been done in which volunteers were given cigarettes with filters of different absorbency. They were not told which type they were smoking. It was found that when smoking a cigarette with a low nicotine content, or with a filter that filtered off a large amount of nicotine, smokers responded by simply taking deeper and more frequent puffs. Even more revealing is the research that showed if volunteers are given an injection of nicotine, they smoke less. So for the hardened smokers, it is undoubtedly the nicotine which puts the kick into cigarettes.

Besides nicotine, what else have you been inhaling in tobacco smoke? There are over 3,000 chemicals known to be present in every puff you inhale, and most of them are doing you no good. Up to 5 per cent of cigarette smoke is carbon monoxide, the same deadly gas that is in car exhaust fumes. Carbon monoxide passes through the lung tissue and is absorbed into the blood. Here it combines with haemoglobin, the pigment in red blood cells that carries oxygen to all parts of the body to keep them alive. Once carbon monoxide has combined with haemoglobin (to form carboxyhaemoglobin), the blood cells can no longer perform their oxygen-carrying function. In some smokers as much as 15 per cent of haemoglobin can be out of action because it is combined with carbon monoxide. It is not surprising that people who have heart trouble worsen their angina with cigarette smoking for the simple reason that it is depriving the heart muscle of life-giving oxygen. There is no doubt that even a healthy person will reduce his or her ability to exercise and play sports because the oxygen-carrying capacity of the lungs is crippled.

The tar in tobacco smoke contains hundreds of different substances, many of which are known to cause cancer in animals. Some of the most notorious are called nitroso compounds. At a concentration of 1 part per billion nitroso compounds are hazardous in food, yet in unburnt *tobacco* they are present in over 2000 parts per billion. There are two kinds of cancer producing chemicals in cigarette smoke. The nitroso compounds are thought to stimulate the *formation* of a cancer and start it off, and many other substances in tobacco smoke are thought to act as cancer promoters and make it grow.

Many of the chemicals in tobacco smoke are simply irritating. They cause the lungs to produce excessive quantities of sticky mucus as protection for the delicate lining of the bronchial tubes and to make the tubes narrow down. Both of these effects mean that the lungs have to work harder to inhale and exhale air efficiently. In more susceptible people there may even be wheezing, the same breathing difficulty which occurs in asthma.

Other harmful substances present in tobacco smoke include ammonia, used in the manufacture of explosives; bleaches such as sink and lavatory cleaners; powerful poisons such as hydrogen cyanide, which reaches concentrations in cigarette smoke more than 150 times those considered to be safe in industry; solvents such as phenol, used in the paint and plastics industry, which is corrosive, poisonous and a severe irritant.

What effect do you think smoking is having on you? Even though you have just read about the various poisonous substances that are contained in tobacco smoke, do you feel that the brand of cigarette you smoke has a low enough concentration of all these chemicals that you are not affected by them? Do you wonder where all these people are who are supposed to die of lung cancer? Do you feel that of all the people who do smoke, few die of lung cancer, and furthermore that the association isn't proven? Do you feel that it can never happen to you? Just how well informed are you about the effects of cigarette smoking?

Do you really think that it is important for your health to give up smoking? To find out if you really do believe this, here are some questions you might ask yourself. You may find on answering them that you have been fooling yourself about the truly harmful effects of smoking on you today.

1 Do you think that cigarette smoking is dangerous enough to do something about it?

2 Do you think that if cigarette smoking were put in a list of health hazards, it would come rather low?

3 Do you think that the health problems caused by cigarette smoking are very minor ones?

If you agree with these propositions, you really are badly informed about the dangerous effects of smoking on health. Here are a few statistics that back up what I say:

1 One in every six deaths is caused by smoking.

2 The death rate among women who smoke is the same as for men who smoke.

3 People who smoke have more illnesses of all kinds than people who don't.

4 One fifth of all time lost from work is because of illness due to cigarette smoking.

5 You may know about the association of cigarette smoking and lung cancer, but life threatening heart disease and crippling chronic bronchitis and emphysema are in many cases, also caused by smoking cigarettes. You can't ignore these risks.

Do you feel that you are an exception to all the statistics? To see if you do ask yourself these questions:

1 Do you think that your brand of cigarette is much less likely to cause diseases associated with cigarette smoking?

2 Do you think that you haven't smoked long enough to have to worry about the diseases caused by cigarette smoking?

3 Do you think you smoke too few cigarettes to be in danger of getting any of the diseases associated with cigarette smoking?

If you agree with these statements, you really do believe that it can't happen to you. You are wrong, and in your heart you know you are, but you haven't faced up to the truth. The thing about cigarette smoking is that even a few cigarettes a day can damage your health. What is more, any of the diseases associated with cigarette smoking can strike you at any time. You don't get any warning, and by the time you come to your senses it may be too late. As you get older your lungs become less capable of over-coming an infection and so any winter cold may turn into pneumonia. No matter how few cigarettes you smoke your risk of dying through any kind of serious illness is greater than average.

Have you tried to stop smoking before and failed? Do you have very little confidence in your ability to stop smoking? To see if this is your attitude ask yourself the following questions:

1 Do you feel that it is just too difficult even to try cutting down on your cigarettes?

2 Do you think that you will always relapse, even if you succeed for two or three weeks in stopping smoking?

3 Do you think that it would be just too difficult for you to make any kind of change in your smoking habits?

4 Do you feel that you've smoked for so long that there is no *point* in giving up?

If you have answered yes to these questions, you really have a low opinion of yourself. Lower than anyone deserves to have. This could be because you have never tackled stopping smoking in a systematic or practical way. Just because you have failed once, doesn't mean to say that you can't succeed the next time. Most smokers who are eventually successful in giving up have tried before and failed, so don't let that put you off. This time you are going to succeed. Nearly 40 million adults in the world have given up smoking successfully. You are going to get a lot of help in Chapter 3 and Chapter 5 where you will be shown how to plan and organise your personal campaign to become an ex-smoker, and this time you will succeed.

Do you think there is little value in giving up smoking? Do you feel there are few benefits to be gained? Try asking yourself these questions:

1 Do you know that a person's body starts to recover from the damage of smoking as soon as they stop?

2 Do you know that a person is likely to live longer if they stop smoking?

3 Do you know that even if you have been smoking for quite a long time anyway, it will do you good to stop?

If you have answered no to most of these questions, then you really haven't thought seriously about the benefits of giving up smoking. The wonderful thing about stopping is that for no matter how long you have smoked, your body starts recovering the moment that you stop. Your lungs can recover from most of the effects of chronic bronchitis. Indeed they start recovering within minutes of being free from cigarette smoke.

But cigarette smoking can damage your lungs to such an extent that they become inelastic and inefficient. When you reach this stage the structural damage to your lungs is irreversible so it is important to stop now. The deleterious effects of smoking, such as increasing breathlessness, the start of wheezing, a cough every morning, a cold every winter, may be so gradual, that you accept them as part of day to day ageing. One day however, you could find yourself so breathless that you are confined to a wheel chair.

Finally if you already have a peptic ulcer, any kind of chest disease, if there is heart disease in the family, if you have had a heart attack already, then you really should give up smoking, because it is so difficult to control any of these diseases if you continue to smoke.

While I was making the BBC Television series *So You Want to Stop Smoking*, Dr Howard Williams introduced me to some of his patients who were suffering from diseases related to smoking. In his chest clinic he sees many people with chronic lung disease, who have smoked for years. Some of them have gone on smoking heavily in the face of chest disease. Some have continued to smoke even after a heart attack, even when they have such severe disease in the leg arteries that a part of a leg has been amputated, or a foot has become gangrenous.

One of the patients I got to know rather well was Mr Petherbridge. He was in his early sixties, and when I first met him sitting up in bed, he looked pink and healthy as though there was very little wrong with him. This was because he was completely at rest, putting no strain on his body. However, when he got out of bed to go to the bathroom it was quite another story. He was breathless with the exertion of having to put on his dressing gown. He had to stop at the end of the next bed and hold on to the rail to catch his breath. From then on he needed a nurse to support him because the slightest exertion made him wheeze. By the time he got to the bathroom, he was a greyish blue colour. He was coughing and he could hardly get his breath for wheezing. Mr Petherbridge suffered from emphysema, a destructive complication of chronic bronchitis.

Mr Petherbridge told me the story of his chest disease and his smoking habits. He had accepted the gradual deterioration in his breathing over many years. He had felt that serious disease due to cigarette smoking was unlikely to happen to him.

He felt that he didn't smoke sufficient cigarettes to get a serious disease from smoking, and so he had continued to smoke. For the past five years he had virtually been a respiratory cripple.

We interviewed Mr Petherbridge for the programme, because he expressed some of the misconceptions about smoking that we felt people could learn from. We showed a chest X-ray of Mr Petherbridge taken a few months earlier, which had a classical picture of diseased lungs obvious even to the untrained eye.

A week or so after filming him, Mr Petherbridge's condition

became markedly worse. He was re-investigated. To my horror, I learned that he had lung cancer. From being a middle-aged man suffering from emphysema, with a *moderately high* risk of a premature death due to a smoking related disease, Mr Petherbridge was plunged into an *extremely high risk* group of people who are likely to die very quickly from a fatal smoking-related disease.

Let's just take a look back on Mr Petherbridge's life and find out what had set him on his fatal course. What was there about his smoking habits that started the slow-burning fuse towards a death from lung cancer before the age of 65? What might he have done at various stages during his life to reduce the risk of getting lung cancer? Could he have avoided the development of lung cancer altogether? What would he have had to do to prevent emphysema from developing? How would he have had to change his lifestyle to keep healthy lungs, to be fit and active and enjoy his middle age and retirement? Could anything have preserved his good health and avoided lung cancer? To try to answer these questions let's see what kind of smoker Mr Petherbridge was.

Like most smokers Mr Petherbridge began to smoke in his early teens. He didn't really enjoy his first cigarette. In fact he didn't enjoy the first half dozen. They made him feel dizzy and sick. After he had smoked about ten cigarettes he learned just the right size of puff to take so that he didn't cough and splutter when he inhaled, and once he had found how much smoke to draw into his lungs to get the amount of nicotine that suited him, he felt a good deal happier.

Even though he didn't enjoy smoking much in the beginning, he persisted, because the group of boys he went around with all smoked and when they smoked as a gang together he felt the odd one out if he didn't. They all used to joke about him not smoking, and poke fun at him. So he was under quite a lot of social pressure to smoke and most of his first cigarettes were smoked with the group-social cigarettes. But it wasn't long before he was wanting to smoke when he was on his own and he very quickly learned the quiet satisfaction of smoking a cigarette in private.

Most people learn to smoke in childhood or adolescence. If you and your children can make it to 20 without smoking you and they probably never will take it up. So it falls to parents – and school teachers – to aim for non smoking teenagers and do everything possible to deter teenagers from starting the habit.

Children from some backgrounds are more at risk of starting to smoke than others. These are the factors that favour smoking:

Here are some pressures which made Mr Petherbridge as a young teenager take up smoking – and could affect your children too. Watch out for them.

- Large number of friends smoke
- Pressure from friends
- Trying to appear grown up
- Boosting self confidence
- Appearing tough (complying with a media image)
- Friends smoking
- Parents smoking
- Brothers and sisters smoking
- Curiosity
- Rebelliousness
- Cigarettes easy to obtain

SMOKER

NON-SMOKER

Had the pressures below been stronger he may never have become a smoker – parents control most of these pressures.

- Boosting of self confidence in the home, being treated as a growing adult
- Pursuit of out-door pleasures
- Encouragement to stay fit to play sports
- Attitudes at school towards smoking
- Knowledge of health risks associated with smoking
- Brothers and sisters don't smoke and don't like it
- Parental attitude to smoking is disapproving
- Parents non-smokers

1 Lower socio-economic class.

2 Parents who smoke.

3 Parents who leave cigarettes lying around the house.

4 Parents who implicitly approve, whatever their own smoking habits.

5 Older brothers and sisters who smoke.

6 Schools where a high proportion of teachers smoke.

A few children smoke their first cigarettes when they are as young as five years old. Approximately 1 in 3 of these is a regular smoker by the age of 9. A third of all boys smoke by the time they're 15, though somewhat fewer girls. As the following picture shows however, more and more girls are smoking cigarettes younger and younger, possibly because the psychological pressures mentioned are still having an increased impact on girls.

By the time he was seventeen, Mr Petherbridge was working in an accountant's office and attending night school to study for exams. He was working quite hard and felt a lot of pressure in the office. It was also quite a strain to be studying in the evening. He quickly found that smoking was relaxing, and also helped him to concentrate when he was studying late at night.

Like many other smokers, Mr Petherbridge was quite an extrovert, very often the life and soul of the party, and his boss in the office said that he would have to become less impulsive and not take so many risks. Also he got a few tellings-off because he was very quick to oppose authority. As a typical young smoker, Mr Petherbridge changed his job a couple of times before settling down, and seemed to have a proneness to car accidents. He was a great tea and coffee drinker as many heavy smokers are.

By the time he was twenty, Mr Petherbridge was smoking automatically without thinking about it and was up to 30 unfiltered cigarettes a day. At this stage, he was fit. He didn't have a smoker's cough in the morning. He didn't suffer from winter colds nor was there a hint of bronchitis. In fact he used to play in the local football team, so he was a strong and healthy young man.

Mr Petherbridge answered a questionnaire for us which gave us quite a clear picture of the kind of smoker he was. Here are some of his answers:

I usually find smoking cigarettes relaxing and pleasant.

Smoking habits in boys and girls

For every 100 youngsters, the number who
were smoking one or more cigarettes a week.

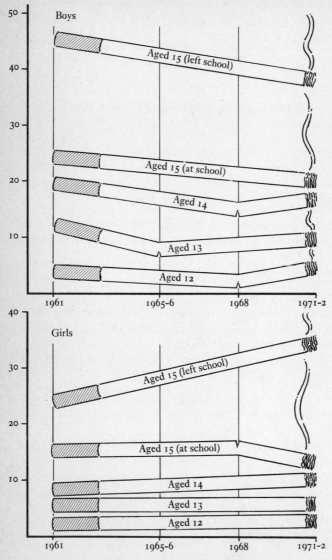

The habit increased in fifteen year old girls once they'd left school,
whereas the opposite happened in boys.

I can't think of any cigarettes in the day which aren't enjoyable.
I smoke cigarettes when—

I am angry.

I feel myself slowing down.

I want to wake myself up.

I need a lift when I am with friends.

I feel relaxed and comfortable.

I feel worried and a bit depressed.

I want to take my mind off things.

The things I like about smoking cigarettes would be:

Watching the smoke as I exhale it.

Feeling the cigarette between my fingers and in my mouth.

The pack of cigarettes and the lighter are attractive.

The ritual of lighting up a cigarette.

I am doing something with my hands.

I must like smoking because:

I sometimes light up two cigarettes at once in different parts of the room without realising it.

I really hate it when I run out of cigarettes and have actually gone out late at night to get a pack from a cigarette machine.

When I don't smoke for a couple of hours, I get a real craving for a cigarette.

Sometimes I find myself smoking a cigarette without remembering having lit it.

When things are bad in the office I count up my cigarettes and find that I have smoked five in the last half hour without realising it.

With a cigarette in my hand I feel complete – I am always aware of *not* smoking one.

This profile of Mr Petherbridge showed him to be the classical heavy smoker. He loved handling cigarettes. He loved the feel of them. Many cultures have devised ways of satisfying this need without smoking cigarettes. In Mediterranean countries worry beads are used. If you find handling cigarettes very pleasureable, it will be easier to give up if:

You keep your hands and fingers occupied with something

small and just as pleasant to hold – a key ring, a small toy, a nice pen or a pencil – or even worry beads, why not?

Mr Petherbridge used smoking as stimulation. If you do too you will find that:

You will get just as much stimulation from moderate exercise such as a brisk walk around the block.
You should consider trying exercise to help you to stop smoking.

Many smokers use cigarettes as emotional support, a crutch when life is stressful. Smoking isn't going to solve problems or make them go away. Even during and after the cigarette the problem remains. If you go on using cigarettes as a crutch, you may find yourself smoking more because they become less effective at relieving the stress. You may find that some of these things act as good substitutes:

Going out and meeting people, keeping yourself occupied, distracting yourself from your worries with any kind of activity – odd jobs around the house, dress making, golf etc. and any kind of physical exercise can act as a better calming agent than a cigarette and it is better for your health all round.

If like Mr Petherbridge, cigarettes help you to relax and feel good, you are probably one of those smokers who gets a great deal of pleasure out of smoking, especially at certain times of the day, like with your mid-morning cup of coffee or after dinner in the evening. If smoking were simply for pleasure, most determined non-smokers would find it quite easy to get a substitute. You can:

Do *anything else* that brings you pleasure, but doesn't have the health risks.

Some of Mr Petherbridge's answers, like his anxiety about running out of cigarettes, show that he is really psychologically addicted to smoking. If you are in the same category, you are probably no longer enjoying smoking. To you it probably seems to be a necessity. It is possible that the craving for a cigarette begins as soon as you put the last one out. One good thing about being this kind of smoker is that if you do initially crack your psychological dependency, you will probably never want to go through the discomfort again. This means that after only a couple of weeks you will be a non-smoker for the rest of your life. You are also someone who responds well to a challenge and will really want to try. Unlikely though it seems there are a lot of things going for you. Because of your kind of dependency there is one thing you should avoid doing:

> Don't try to stop smoking by *reducing* your cigarette intake. You are going to have to do it 'Cold Turkey'. You will have to choose a day, smoke your last cigarette and stop. Your particular problem is going to be a craving for cigarettes especially at the times of day when you enjoyed them most so you are going to have to plan and prepare yourself very well (see page 54). However, remember, the really bad cravings last no longer than a few minutes so that is all you have to get through, and there are many simple ways of doing that (see page 52). You can get yourself through most cravings by drinking a glass of water, sucking a peppermint, changing your surroundings and immersing yourself in an activity which demands all of your concentration.

If you are smoking automatically like Mr Petherbridge, then smoking has become a habit and brings you little real pleasure. If you ever light up a cigarette without realising that you still have another burning in the ash tray you are in this group. What you are going to have to do is to break your habits. Most cigarette smoking habits are associated with certain activities and certain places, so the things you should be thinking about doing this week are:

1 Changing your habits, changing your routine and changing your environment.

2 Not having coffee in the middle of the morning, having fruit juice instead.

3 Having tea if you normally have coffee after your evening meal.

4 Not sitting at the table after the meal.

5 Going to the non-smoking part of restaurants, buses and trains.

6 Sitting next to a non-smoker at a meeting.

7 Leaving your cigarettes behind when you go out on a job etc.

As far as Mr Petherbridge's health risks are concerned, let's take a look at some of the risks he was running when he was twenty and smoking 30 unfiltered cigarettes a day. You can get an idea

Your risk of death related to the age you start to smoke

Deaths in a year for every 1,000 men

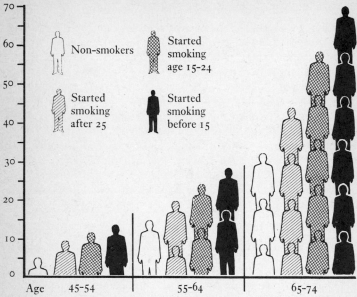

of how much he would have lowered his risk by giving up smoking if you compare his health risks with those of a non-smoker aged twenty. In fact, the figures shown are for 10–19 cigarettes a day, and Mr Petherbridge smoked many more than this. Of course you must remember that death-rates increase with age. But even after taking that into account, in every age group the death rate is higher for those people who started to smoke at an earlier age. So if we take the 45–54 age group Mr Petherbridge, even if he had only smoked 19 cigarettes a day, would have fallen into a group of people whose death rate was about 15 per 1000. Whereas if he'd never smoked he would have been in a group where the chances of dying were about five in a thousand. In other words, by smoking he had tripled his chance of dying even as early as when he was 45 or 50 years old.

If we try to estimate how much Mr Petherbridge could have increased his life expectancy by stopping smoking look at the age range 55–64. When he entered this group, Mr Petherbridge was among people in whom the death is more than 20 in 1000. As the body recovers very quickly from the effects of smoking, if there is no permanent damage to the lungs, we could say that Mr Petherbridge would have cut his risk by almost half if he'd become a non-smoker.

Your chances of drying from Lung Cancer related to how heavily you smoke

Increase in risk of dying

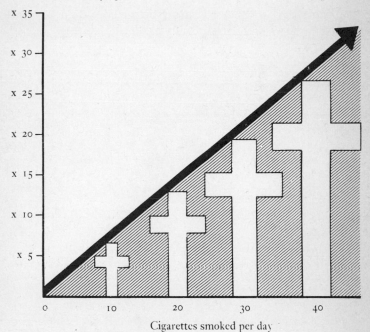

Cigarettes smoked per day

If Mr Petherbridge had cut down the number of cigarettes he was smoking per day when he was 20 he could have greatly reduced his chances of getting lung cancer. This pictures shows that the more you smoke, the more chances you stand of developing lung cancer.

At 20, Mr Petherbridge was smoking 30 cigarettes a day. As far back as that he had a 15 times greater chance of getting lung cancer than a non-smoker. If only he'd cut down to 10 a day his chances would have been reduced to a 5 times risk. So at twenty, he lost the opportunity to give himself three times the chance of staying alive! Remember:

1 You are not immune.

2 If you smoke 15 to 25 cigarettes a day you have a 1 in 8 chance of developing lung cancer.

3 If you are smoking 25 or more cigarettes a day your chances are 1 in 5.

If you are comforting yourself with the old chestnut that you stand a greater chance of dying crossing the road, you are wrong.

4 Smoking causes 7 times as many premature deaths as road accidents.

3 Deciding to stop

You may have tried to stop smoking before and failed. That doesn't mean that you will fail this time. This time, you are going to be successful, so try again. You can be successful, even if you are a heavy smoker and even if you started to smoke in your early teens. This time you will have the help and support of this book, and you will have a carefully worked out plan to help you to stop, a plan which has proven to be successful in the BBC Television series *So You Want to Stop Smoking*.

Finding the resolve to stop smoking and deciding to do so, is the first and most important step that you will take towards becoming a non-smoker. Most of us make important decisions in steps. The decision to stop smoking is important enough for you to consider as many aspects of it as possible. If you think through all your concerns, you will feel confident and you will increase your resolve. You will be better equipped to deal with difficulties and you will increase your chances of success. One aspect of the decision that you must not overlook is *how* you are going to stop smoking. It is essential that you choose a way which is easiest for you and suits your personality. (There are several ways you can go about it, all of which are dealt with in Chapter 9). This is a resume for you to think about while you are preparing to stop.

You can decide to smoke your last cigarette and then no more – Cold Turkey. Many people find this the easiest way. It's a clean break. It's a new way of life. You're starting something new. You may decide on a new hair style too, or a new suit of clothes. Even though this is the way you have decided to stop smoking you may not be able to make the decision about *when* immediately, so don't. You don't have to. But you have to decide some day in the very near future. Don't back off from the decision. *When* you stop is important so give it some thought. Don't stop during the week, if you smoke at the office. The weekend is a bad time to stop if you smoke to relax when work's over. So make it easy on yourself. If a birthday or anniversary is coming up that could be a good time, once you've decided. Mark it clearly in your diary and on every calendar around the house, because it is 'D' Day.

Another way, though it is not one that I endorse, is to reduce the number of cigarettes you smoke until you are smoking four or five a day and then gradually stop. You are weaning yourself off nicotine. But be warned. This is a fairly difficult way to stop smoking, possibly because you are merely putting off the evil day when you have to go without cigarettes completely. If you have tried this method before and failed, it is better not to use it. Most experts in the field of smoking cessation, would not recommend this approach.

Many smokers are stimulated to give up when they realise that smoking has such a grip on them that they have unconsciously smoked as many as sixty or eighty in one day. They are filled with such a feeling of self-loathing that it carries them through the first few days of stopping smoking. You can devise a programme to 'disgust' yourself into giving up. This is a kind self-imposed aversion therapy and can be quite successful, though you shouldn't attempt it without your doctor's approval. It has proven most rewarding in the hands of specialists who get you to inhale deeply every six seconds until you feel sick and can take no more. As soon as you feel better you repeat the whole routine, three or four times in 30 minutes, at which point you may feel so awful you pack in smoking there and then. If not you repeat the programme, the next day and the next until smoking is so awful you can't go on.

For those of you who like a set of rules to follow, there is a method that involves just that. Furthermore you can write your own rules. That doesn't mean being easy on yourself. In fact most people are quite the opposite. They set themselves fairly strict rules. In writing them you are making a contract with yourself to obey them and never break them. The attractive thing about this method is that you can start off with fairly manageable rules and then as you stick to them successfully you can make them more difficult. These are examples of some of the rules you might decide you are going to stick to:

1 Never smoke in the car.
2 Only start smoking when nearly at your destination.
3 Refuse every cigarette that is offered to you.
4 Stop smoking before a meal.
5 Don't have a cigarette before breakfast.

6 Only buy one packet of cigarettes at a time.

7 Only buy ten cigarettes instead of twenty.

8 Buy a different brand of cigarettes every time, not just your favourite.

9 Before you light a cigarette count to ten.

10 Every time you take a cigarette, put the pack away at a distance from where you are, in another room if possible.

11 When you run out of cigarettes, never take one from someone else.

12 After each puff put the cigarette down.

13 Never smoke out of doors.

14 Never smoke in bed.

15 Stop smoking at work.

16 Stop smoking in the house.

17 Stop carrying your lighter or matches with you so that you have to ask for a light.

18 Stop smoking when you are using your hands for something else.

19 Stop inhaling.

20 Stop smoking a cigarette more than half way down.

21 Stop smoking after a meal while you are sitting at the table. Wait until you have gone into another room.

22 Stop smoking while you are waiting for something. A phone call. Waiting for the bus, another person.

23 When you are smoking stop doing anything else – for instance having a cup of coffee, a drink, watching television, listening to music etc.

24 Stop smoking if someone lights up in your presence. Don't smoke during working hours.

25 Don't smoke while you are relaxing after work with a drink.

26 Only smoke if you are sitting in an uncomfortable chair.

27 Keep a rubber-band round your cigarette pack so you are aware of opening it.

28 Time your smoking frequency. Have a cigarette on the hour. Then try every other hour.

Don't start obeying all of these rules on the first day. You should choose three or four, never more to begin with. If you want to, choose those which seem the easiest to achieve. Success breeds success. Once you have mastered them, add one or two more each day. When you get to the point where you are obeying all the rules, you will have stopped. Dr Brengelmann from Cologne in West Germany devised these rules, and has found that they help people who need discipline. You can be a little tough on yourself if you want to, imposing a fine should you break a rule. If you break a rule once, that doesn't mean that you have to give up. You fine yourself, put some money in the 'Quit Kitty', and carry on. You can make it easier on yourself with a reward if you find that you have stuck to the rules for one day. After a week you could buy yourself a small present.

The results of keeping a smoking diary of *when* you smoked, *why* you smoked, and *how much* you wanted to smoke, will have given you quite a lot of information about yourself and your smoking habits. Like most smokers who keep a cigarette diary you will have found that the majority of them weren't really needed. It should be fairly easy to pin-point the cigarettes you feel you can't do without. These are the ones that are going to be difficult to give up. Most people are remarkably alike when it comes to the most important cigarettes of the day, and here are some of them:

The first cigarette of the day

Most smokers want a cigarette shortly after waking up. For some it is the first thing they do. They reach for the packet of cigarettes which are kept by the bed. Others have one within a few minutes of getting up with the first cup of coffee or cup of tea before breakfast. Very few smokers wait to eat before their first cigarette. Many smokers say that the first cigarette is the best cigarette of the day. It tastes very good because the nicotine level in the blood has dropped during the night. Many people say that it wakes them up and the first few deep draws on the cigarette can make them feel quite dizzy.

If you wait until breakfast time to have your first cigarette, this can be quite a hard one for you to give up, because it punctuates the day, it starts it off. For many people, breakfast consists of nothing else other than a cup of tea or coffee with a cigarette. If you fall into either of these cases you are going to have to think of things to distract yourself, or you are going to have to change your early morning routine, so that going without that first cigarette doesn't seem so bad.

The cigarette while travelling to work

If you have to travel any distance, be it by rail or by road, many people find that a cigarette on the way to work, acts as a preparation for the day ahead. It may make them feel more alert and it calms the nerves after the hectic rush, to get up have breakfast and dash out of the house.

The stress cigarette

Most people meet a problem shortly after getting to work. A smoker's reaction is to reach for a cigarette. You may automatically search for the packet as you go through the mail, get your desk straight, or as soon as the telephone rings. The habit of reaching for a cigarette as soon as you feel anxious, worried, or pressured is something which will continue throughout the day.

The coffee break cigarette

This is one of the commonest rituals of all. Nearly everyone who smokes feels that a cigarette is inseparable from a cup of coffee or a cup of tea at break time. It helps to pass the time. It helps to define the break more clearly. It is relaxing, even soothing, and has been shown to be stimulating. Many smokers find that they have more energy after the 'break' cigarette.

The telephone cigarette

Another common ritual is automatically lighting a cigarette as soon as the telephone rings and smoking while answering it. This ritual can become so ingrained that it is almost impossible to have a telephone conversation without a cigarette and smokers often ask the caller to hang on while they find one. This cigarette is usually smoked for its calming effect and also because it seems to concentrate the mind. It also gives you a pause to think if you are asked questions or for information.

The before and after-work cigarette

Many people find that they like to have a cigarette as soon as work is ended. So they have one just before going to lunch, when lunch is over and they are about to start on the afternoon stint, and when work is over in the evening. This is another 'Ritual' cigarette which is clearly associated with a specific activity. It is this kind of cigarette where you're going to have to break the ritual or take steps to avoid it if you're going to conquer the habit.

The working cigarette

If you have decided that there is a particular job to be done, and you have made preparations to do it, and you are all set to start, the temptation is to reach for a cigarette, as an accompaniment to your activity. Many smokers enjoy these cigarettes because they become associated with the satisfaction of a job well done, or difficult problems solved. Smokers may think that they couldn't have done the job or solved the problems without the cigarette. Of course this is not true.

The cigarette when work is over for the day

Around about 6.30 or 7 o'clock, whether having a drink with colleagues after work or at home, it is a very common ritual to light up a cigarette. It tells you that the work day is over. It is time to relax, and you usually settle down in your favourite armchair with a drink or a cup of tea, make yourself comfortable and gradually wind down. This is also an attractive cigarette, because the sensations and the associations are so pleasurable.

The cigarette after dinner

Anyone who has given up smoking will probably confess that this is the hardest cigarette of all to give up. Smokers who have been non-smokers for many years, confess that occasionally after dinner, they still feel like having a cigarette with their coffee. Their desire is rarely strong enough to be called a craving. This cigarette can also be difficult to give up because it is part and parcel of enjoying good food and convivial company.

The evening cigarette

Whatever you do during the evening after work and dinner, if it is reading the newspaper or a book, listening to music, or watching TV, a cigarette is often part of the relaxation. Any cigarette which is associated with feelings of pleasure, and lack of tension is going to be hard to give up.

The cigarette before going to sleep

The last cigarette of the day is also one of the most enjoyable.

This is usually a contemplative cigarette where you think what has happened during the day, what is to be done tomorrow. It is also a calming cigarette, and it makes you feel tranquil and ready for sleep.

The middle of the night cigarette

If you are having difficulty sleeping, you may well switch on the light and reach for a cigarette in the middle of the night in the hope that it will make you calm enough to go back to sleep.

Tips and guidelines of how to deal with all these difficult cigarettes are given further on in the book.

Once you have decided to stop smoking you must make your decision public. Tell your partner, all the members of your family, your colleagues and the people that you meet frequently that you are going to stop smoking. You should also encourage them to support you by not offering you cigarettes and by not discouraging you. Letting people know you mean business and are prepared to put some effort into stopping will help you take your decision seriously yourself.

In your own home you have to ask your family to do a little more. Ask your partner to be supportive and encourage you. Make an agreement that they are not going to do anything to weaken your resolve. If they smoke and are not going to give up with you, ask them not to smoke in the same room as you, not to leave cigarettes lying around and not to make cigarettes the subject of conversations. You should also ask for their help by substituting covered ash trays for open ones so that you can't smell cigarettes, and never offering you one or discouraging you. The best kind of support is your partner giving up with you. Two resolves are stronger than one, and a bit of competition between you not to fail is all to the good. If your partner won't join you, don't be deterred, but you might suggest that they join you in a 'contract' to help you to stop smoking (see page 41).

You should decide that stopping smoking will not be an excuse for putting on weight. You need to plan ahead. Give quite a lot of thought to your diet, and part of your decision to stop should be a decision not to gain weight. If you decide to do this you will have dealt with one of the greatest worries that people have about giving up smoking. Many people feel that putting on weight is inescapable if they give up smoking. They feel that they will eat more and nibble more. Nibbles are nearly always high calorie foods since those are the foods that are most readily available.

You have to prepare yourself to eat a good diet, resist high calorie nibbles and substitute healthy low calorie snack foods.

There is no evidence that stopping smoking will increase your craving for rich foods, sweets and chocolates. It does not. Appetite may well improve and food may probably taste better, but you don't have to substitute chocolate for cigarettes. If you have any concerns about putting on weight when you stop smoking then you should decide now how you are going to avoid it. There are several things you can do. One of the stoppers in the BBC series *So You Want to Stop Smoking* took the very intelligent precaution of losing seven pounds in weight before she ever stopped smoking, so that she didn't have to worry so much about what she was eating, and could concentrate all her efforts on stopping smoking. She had seven pounds to play with during the first few difficult weeks. You might try doing the same thing.

Another thing to do is to keep a daily diary for a week of what you normally eat, noting each food and the quantity you eat at every meal. After about a week you will have a very good idea of what your normal eating habits are, and you can calculate roughly how many calories you take in per day. Once you have stopped smoking you can continue to count calories and make sure – even though you do take a few nibbles during the day – that you don't exceed your normal calorie intake. Calorie counting has the advantage that it is very flexible. If you want to you can nibble at the odd biscuit (make sure it is Rich Tea, they are the lowest in calories), or have a bar of chocolate if that is what you particularly want to do as long as you go without something later on in the day so that you don't exceed your calorie quota.

You can decide to change your eating habits so that you eat a good balanced diet with very little of the empty calorie foods, such as sweets, chocolates, cakes and biscuits, jams, rich sauces, cream etc., and you should do this well before stopping smoking.

If all of these things seem a little hard for you and you feel that you can't cope with being careful about your food as well as stopping smoking for heavens sake concentrate on stopping smoking. Even though there are stories of large weight gains in people who are stopping smoking, it is rare rather than the rule. Research has shown that the majority of smokers who do gain weight put on no more than a few pounds. Don't worry about it too much. Anyone who can conquer smoking, can always manage to lose a few pounds in weight.

If you smoke to relax and feel that you will never be able to give up the cigarettes that help you to cope with stress, then one of the things you have to decide to do is to manage your stress and teach yourself to relax. You can do both of them without cigarettes (see pages 59–64).

Contract to stop smoking

Signing a contract to stop smoking may seem to be going a bit far, but it works. Many studies have shown that people who enter into contracts with a supporter or helper when they are trying to break a habit or change their behaviour stand a much greater chance of success than trying to do it alone. Many studies have shown that there are certain rules to this game.

1 The contract should be for six months, but three months at the least. In other words you enter into the contract not to smoke for six months and your helper enters into the contract for the same length of time.

2 Neither you nor your helper can break the contract. You will find this easier to adhere to if you have an independent referee.

3 Make sure that the person with whom you take out your contract is as determined as you are. Avoid making a contract with someone who may put temptation your way.

4 The contracts should be so arranged that if you relapse, both of you pay a high price. You might decide for instance that the two of you will make quite a large contribution to an organisation that you both dislike very much.

Your contract could be something like this:

```
I HAVE DECIDED TO GIVE UP SMOKING.  I will undertake all of
these actions:

  1  I will decide HOW I'm going to stop smoking.


  2  I will decide WHEN I'm going to stop smoking and mark it in
     my diary.


  3  I will make my decision public and tell my family, friends
     and people I work with that I am quitting.  I will try to
     get their support.


  4  I will check my weight and plan a balanced diet if I think
     I'll gain weight.  I'll start buying low calorie nibbles.
```

5   I will study and practice one method of relaxing and one method of stress control as outlined in Chapter 5 of this book.

6   I will decide which are my most difficult cigarettes of the day and PREPARE to stop smoking by reading Chapter 5 of this book.

7   I shall seek help from (insert name of partner or friend) who will encourage me at all times to be a non-smoker, and whom I can call on at all times for support.

8   I shall read all of the rest of this book and re-read it if my morale needs boosting. I will carry it with me at all times.

9   I shall stop smoking finally on (date).

10 When I have not smoked for six months myself and ....
    will reward ourselves with .... (fill in rewards)

11 If I fail to give up smoking I and ....
    will not only forfeit our rewards but will each pay the
    sum of £50 to ....

N.B. I will (rather than I shall) means I promise.

Signed................(Non-smoker) Signed...... ....(Sponsor)

Witnessed .... Witnessed ....

Date .... Date ....

4 Hard Facts II

Smoking and Your Everyday Health

There is hardly a smoker for whom the quality of life is not the poorer for smoking. Nearly every smoker lives with at least one detrimental effect of smoking. You may be unaware of it, because the damaging effects of smoking are insidious. They creep up on you gradually and their progress may be so slow that from month to month and even year to year you do not realise how much your health is deteriorating.

The smoker's cough (which has erroneously been called the morning cough – may be worst in the morning, but it often persists all day), is one of the first signs that smoking is irritating your lungs, and damaging them. Chemicals in the tar fraction of cigarette smoke cause several deleterious things to happen in the lungs. First of all they injure the surface of the air passages, in very much the same way as cigarette smoke makes the eyes sting and produce tears to get rid of chemicals in the smoke. The lungs don't produce tears. They produce phlegm to wash away the irritant. Substances in cigarette smoke paralyse the cilia, microscopic hairs on the surface of the bronchial tubes which waft particles of dust and grime up to the throat to be coughed out. Cilia are constantly sweeping the lungs clean. Other substances in the smoke cause the cells to lose their healthy appearance. Instead of being plump, they become thin and flat and this is one of the first changes seen when a cell is on its way to becoming a cancer.

The smoker's cough is typically present all the year round regardless of season. But during the winter differences between smokers and non-smokers become really apparent. It is thought that substances in cigarette smoke damage the body's immunological responses, thereby making it less able to resist infections. For this reason cigarette smokers suffer from more colds than non-smokers and they go on and on for weeks. Smokers frequently complain that a head cold ends up as sinisitus, requiring a long course of antibiotics to eradicate it. Then winter colds start to go down on to the chest and cause bronchitis. This is the first step on the road to chronic bronchitis, but many smokers don't seem to mind these minor illnesses. I didn't when I was a smoker.

Damage to the lungs can begin quite early. A teenager who smokes more than five cigarettes a week may cough as much and produce as much excess phlegm as a smoker who has smoked for years. The smokers who do the most damage to themselves are those who inhale most, make their own roll-ups, smoke unfiltered cigarettes, and always have a cigarette in the corner of their mouths, probably because they breathe in the side stream of unfiltered smoke which is a good deal more irritating than filtered smoke. If you are a smoker who suffers from a smoker's cough, never seems to be able to get rid of a cold in the winter, or expects a cold to go on to your chest, then smoking is really damaging your health and for your own sake you should stop.

The marvellous news about stopping smoking is that the very minute you stop your lungs begin to recover and heal themselves. You prevent damage from going any further. However once you have signs of lung damage, the greater the damage will become and the more irreversible it is if you continue to smoke.

The next phase in the development of chronic bronchitis is narrowing of the bronchial tubes, and you may notice wheezing. At first it may be only when you get a cold or bronchitis, but it will become more frequent. Once the bronchial tubes are narrowed, the lungs are deprived of a good supply of fresh air and oxygen and the rest of the body cannot be properly nourished. The lungs have to do more work to get the required quantity of air in and out of the lungs. Not only do the lungs suffer but the heart suffers from this poor oxygen supply, and it has to work harder, so it is under strain.

One of the later stages of chronic bronchitis is emphysema. The irritation caused by cigarette smoke may be so severe that the microscopic air spaces, the alveoli, burst forming large air spaces in the lungs. This makes the passage of oxygen into the blood, and carbon dioxide out of the blood, even less efficient. People with emphysema find any kind of exercise too difficult to undertake. They may get breathless walking as short a distance as across a room. Quite often they are confined to bed or a wheel chair, and may only be able to move by crawling on their hands and knees.

Every smoker is on the slippery slope to emphysema. Preventing emphysema is one of the best and most important reasons to stop smoking. If you don't you will not only live a shorter life, but your life will be unpleasant while you are living it, and your death will be a lingering and painful one. You will also cause a great deal of suffering to those around you. You only have to look at the immediate future to know that smoking is reducing your physical fitness, and is causing you many irritating minor health problems which you are telling yourself to ignore. Those illnesses however, are enough to account for 50 million lost working days per year in Great Britain.

It has been known for a long time that smoking impairs athletic performance, largely because it interferes with the healthy functioning of the heart and lungs. Because there is carbon monoxide gas dissolved in the blood of smokers, the lungs can neither perform their job of picking up oxygen, nor can the blood transport the oxygen to the muscles when it is needed during muscular exertion. The heart works ineffectively too, and even though athletes who smoke can improve through training, they are always at a disadvantage compared to non-smokers who are going through the same training. Why put yourself at this proven disadvantage?

Smoking is damaging your general health in several other ways. Gingivitis (inflammation of the gums), dental decay and loss of teeth are commoner in people who smoke than those who don't. Oral hygiene tends to be of a lower standard in smokers.

The list of conditions which have been attributed to smoking include loss of hearing, hives (nettle rash) and dermatitis.

The relationship between smoking and peptic ulcers, both duodenal and gastric is well established. In men a peptic ulcer is approximately twice as common amongst smokers than non-smokers, and almost the same in women. While it hasn't been shown conclusively that cigarette smoking increased the production of acid by the stomach, it has been shown that pancreatic juices which neutralise stomach acid are lower when a cigarette is smoked.

The statistics however, are incontrovertible. Eight out of every ten people with a peptic ulcer smoke cigarettes. Smoking delays healing of peptic ulcers. If you stop smoking there's a 70% chance of your ulcer healing *without any treatment*. If you smoke the chances of healing drop to 30%.

If you're a woman, the more you smoke the earlier you are likely to have your menopause, possibly because nicotine can reduce levels of oestrogen, a female hormone. Only 50% of non-smoking women have had a menopause between the ages of 44 and 53 whereas if you smoke 20 or more cigarettes a day you have only a 1 in 3 chance of not having had your menopause. Taking an oral contraceptive pill may slightly increase your chances of having a heart attack, but taking the pill *and* smoking increases your chances 40 times over a non-smoker non-pill taker.

Undoubtedly one of the greatest hazards that you have to contend with if you are a smoker is the possibility of chest complications after a surgical operation which requires a general anaesthetic. If you have an emergency operation, chest complications are almost unavoidable, and doctors will be on the look out for the development of pneumonia after your operation. If on the other hand you have time to prepare for your operation, one of the greatest services you can do for yourself is to cut down your smoking and if possible stop several weeks before you go into hospital.

Cigarette smoking is undoubtedly shortening your life. The most impressive evidence of this belief was gathered here in England in a now world-famous study of British doctors. The study showed that the proportion of men who will die prematurely before retirement (65 years) is 40% for heavy smokers (25 cigarettes or more a day) compared with only 15% for non-smokers.

It is now possible to calculate the number of years of life which a smoker may lose because of the number of cigarettes that he or she is smoking each day. It is even possible to calculate how much your life is shortened, with each cigarette that you smoke. Someone who is smoking 20 cigarettes a day shortens their life by about five years. Even if you are smoking fewer, on average, your life is shortened 5½ minutes for each cigarette smoked – which is about the time you take to smoke it. So when you light up, you not only light up a cigarette, you are lighting a fuse which will explode and shorten your life sooner than need be.

Improving the quality of your life in one step

For anyone who is seriously contemplating giving up smoking, the benefits alone that you will enjoy as the result of your decision make it worthwhile. Think about each one of these benefits for several minutes as you read them over, and if you find your good resolutions weakening, refresh your memory by reading them again. Think about them each day as often as you can remember.

1 Your breath will no longer smell of stale smoke.

2 You will enjoy food more, partly because it tastes better, but also because you have a real appetite for the first time in years (this doesn't mean you have to gain weight. See page 65).

3 Your smokers' cough will disappear.

4 Your breathing will become easier. You won't get breathless with minor exertion.

5 You can really get fit again and play a sport.

6 You can go walking, hiking, swimming, play tennis with the children and family once more.

7 Your fingers and teeth will no longer be stained with nicotine.

8 Your clothes and hair won't smell any more.

9 The car will smell sweeter.

10 The house will smell sweeter.

11 The house and the office and the bedroom will be free of messy ash trays, look more pleasant and be cleaner.

12 Your body will be healing itself every minute. The lungs will no longer produce an excessive amount of phlegm to get rid of smoke particles. That is why your smoker's cough will go. More important, those cells which have become flattened will be growing normally again.

13 You are going to live longer.

14 You are going to be fitter and more active.

15 You will lower your risk of getting bronchitis, emphysema, peptic ulceration, cancer of the lung and heart disease.

16 You are living 5½ minutes longer for every cigarette you don't smoke.

17 You will be saving money. At the current price of cigarettes for someone who smokes a pack a day you are saving nearly £400 per year. This is possibly more than the pay rise you get.

18 You will be setting a good example to others, particularly your children.

19 You should be feeling rather proud of yourself for conquering your habit because it is a real achievement, so your self-esteem will have gone up.

20 You are likely to suffer from fewer colds, and when you do get a cold it will clear up a lot more quickly than it used to just like any other non-smoker.

21 Colds are less likely to go down to your chest or cause sinusitis.

22 You will get a sense of pride every time you say 'No thanks I don't smoke', go into the non-smoking compartment on a train or cinema and join the non-smokers.

23 You have made it much less likely that your children will smoke.

24 If you are pregnant you will have ensured a healthier baby.

25 If you are a singer or an actor or just enjoy using your voice, your voice will have improved.

26 If you have had trouble with your circulation you will feel the cold less.

27 You will be able to wear contact lenses for longer.

28 You will be more attractive.

The continuing story of Mr Petherbridge

Mr Petherbridge is now 30, and he is smoking between 30 and 35 cigarettes a day. He has a smokers' cough in the morning and coughs up quite a lot of phlegm. Two or three years ago he noticed that his colds no longer cleared up, but seemed to drag on for a month or so, and last year his winter cold which he has begun to accept as normal gave him a very nasty attack of bronchitis. He was off work for a couple of weeks and had to take a course of antibiotics. He isn't breathless, but he doesn't play football any more, although he is still interested in the game and quite often referees for the junior team. But he finds even doing that is difficult to keep up. He has heard that a cough is commoner in smokers who smoke untipped cigarettes (and he is right) and so he has changed his brand to filter tips. There is no chronic bronchitis in the family and so he feels protected to some extent by his good constitution. He is quite wrong. The liability to chest disease is more dependent on the number of cigarettes that you smoke than your family history. Tests on identical twins with different smoking habits have shown that there are more chest symptoms and poorer lung function in the twin who smokes more heavily.

Even at this early age, Mr Petherbridge's chance of developing bronchitis is much greater than someone of the same age who doesn't smoke.

Chronic Bronchitis in smokers and non-smokers even where air pollution is high

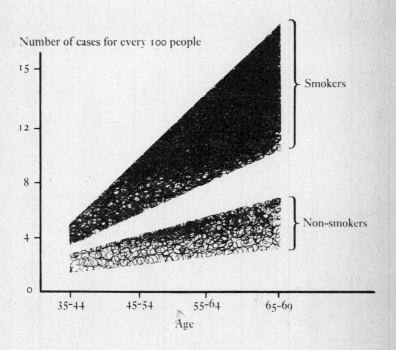

Mr Petherbridge is about to become a statistic. He is entering a group of men who when they reach the age of 35, will only have six chances out of ten of living to see their retirement. If he could stop smoking he would increase his chances to eight out of ten. As he is smoking more than 20 cigarettes a day, he is shortening his life by more than five years. The improvement in Mr Petherbridge's chances of living out his normal life if he stopped smoking now, could be compared to the fall in death rate recorded here for male doctors, as compared to men in general.

Lung Cancer in doctors compared to other men

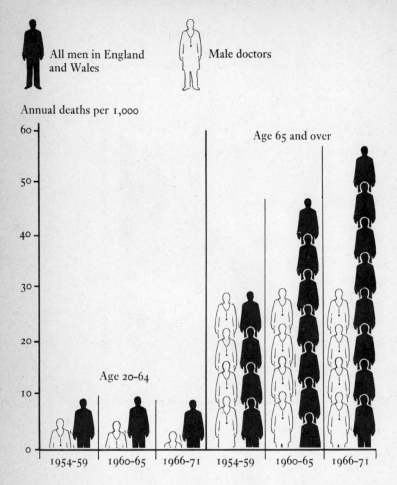

All men in England and Wales

Male doctors

Annual deaths per 1,000

Age 65 and over

Age 20-64

1954-59 1960-65 1966-71 1954-59 1960-65 1966-71

If Mr Petherbridge stopped smoking now, he would move into quite a different statistical group with a much greater chance of life expectancy. In this UK study which looked at the effects of smoking and stopping smoking on doctors, the death rate fell by 22% in doctors under the age of 65 but only by 7% in men of all ages, and this difference was entirely due to diseases associated with smoking. Deaths in all men *rose* by 12% due to diseases associated with smoking, but fell by 26% in doctors.

The death-rate for doctors from any disease compared to other men

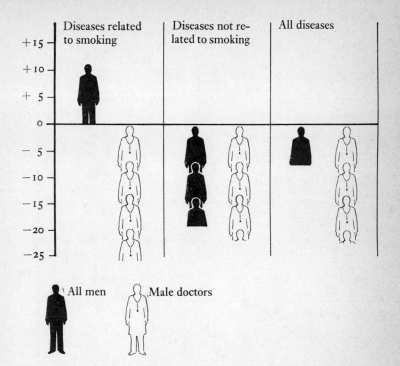

Unknown to himself Mr Petherbridge had entered yet another statistical group – those people who have more general illness, more absence from work due to sickness and attend the doctor more often than the general population. As Mr Petherbridge smokes more than 20 cigarettes a day, he is likely to lose about twice as much time from work as someone who didn't smoke. Compared to a non-smoker, he makes consistently greater use of the medical services at home, in his doctor's surgery, in his doctor's outpatient department and in the hospital ward, so as a smoker he is costing the tax payer a great deal of money in the burden that he puts on the health service.

Crave page

If you feel that your decision to stop smoking is wavering in the next few days here are some things you can do:–

1 Re-read Chapter three.

2 Re-read this Chapter.

3 Re-read the contract you've made with yourself and a friend/ sponsor.

4 Telephone or see your friend/sponsor.

5 Think of your reward if you succeed.

6 Think of your penalty if you fail.

7 Telephone or speak to any non-smoker you know especially if they've given up.

8 Ask your District Health Authority if there's a smoking cessation self-help group in your neighbourhood and talk to them.

5 Preparing to stop

Nearly everyone agrees that *preparing* to stop smoking is one of the best ways you can help yourself and greatly improves your chances of success. If you have tried to stop smoking before and failed, think back to how you tried to stop. Very few people prepare themselves properly for such a radical change of behaviour and if they do, it is usually by accident. Research in smoking cessation clinics all over the world have shown that good preparation for giving up the habit, or rather breaking it, is extremely important.

Preparing, means making a plan. Not just any plan, but a plan that suits *you*. Preparation takes effort. In this chapter, I am going to ask you to do a lot of thinking and then to act. Of all the weeks in the programme this is probably the one where you are going to *do* the most. In doing some of the things I suggest, you're well on the way to becoming a non-smoker. Your programme has started. It is crucial that the plan you prepare is tailor made for you, and no-one else. There is no point in making a plan to stop smoking that you know you can't stick to. Your individual plan has to capitalise on your own particular strengths, and it has to take account of your weaknesses and foibles. We are going to use your strengths and cover your weaknesses.

How smoking is linked to times and places

There are really only two ways of breaking the links. You can either *avoid* the situations where you usually smoke, by trying to break the habit, or you can *fight off* the temptation.

Having kept a diary of all the cigarettes that you smoke during a day, you know very well that you can do without most of them. But the worst ones you are going to have to avoid or fight. Here are some of the ways that you can avoid or fight your most difficult cigarette by either changing the situation in which you usually smoke them, or by overcoming the temptation.

The first cigarette of the day

Breaking the habit

1 Change your waking up routine completely. If you have a teas-made by the bed to wake you up, stop using it so that you have to go downstairs to get your first cup of coffee. This way you will be breaking your routine.

2 Distract yourself with some kind of activity. Switch on the radio if you don't usually listen to it early in the morning. Go downstairs and get the paper if it is delivered early. You might even walk round to the corner shop instead of having it delivered.

3 Make an entirely new rule about your breakfast time ritual. For instance that you will read thrcc pagcs of the newspaper before you go, or that you look up the television programmes to see what is on that evening and mark the ones that you want to see.

Fighting the temptation

1 If you have your first cigarette with a cup of tea or coffee, then substitute fruit juice. Cigarettes really don't taste very pleasant with fresh fruit juice or fruit.

2 Change your breakfast habit altogether so that it helps you to cope with temptation. Spoil yourself at breakfast. Have something that you really like. Change the brand of jam you have. Boil an egg. This will take up time and keep you active and take your mind off smoking.

3 If you have to have a hot drink make it something entirely new like Oxo, Bovril or hot chocolate.

The cigarette while travelling to work

Breaking the habit

1 Make a rule that there is no smoking in the car.

2 If you travel on a bus or a train, go into the non-smoking section.

3 You will notice that the car, bus, train is cleaner, smells fresher, and don't the people really look healthier?

Fighting temptation

1 If you drive to work, try to arrange that you pick up a non-smoking friend, so that you can chat on the way to work, or start listening to the radio or put your favourite tape into the car so that you can listen to your favourite music.

2 If you travel on the bus or the train, make a rule that you are going to read the paper from beginning to end, or that you will start a good book that you have been putting off for ages and that you will read part of it on each of your journeys.

3 If you work close to home, walk to work.

The stress cigarette

Breaking the habit

We can't eradicate stress from our lives, so the best way of coping with it is to control it. This way the need for cigarettes is diminished. When you can control your stress, you can certainly control your need for a cigarette to get you through a stressful patch. How to manage and control stress is dealt with later on in this chapter (see page 59).

Fighting temptation

Even if we are very good at controlling stress, most of us can't control it all the time. In these situations take one minute at a time. Just tell yourself that you will not smoke for a minute. Having got through one minute tackle the next. Think of your success. You have actually gone without a cigarette for sixty seconds and you can do it for another sixty. Take it minute by minute. Once you have managed for five minutes, you should be feeling pretty pleased with yourself, and that would give you the strength to carry on for another five. This way you will see yourself through the stressful patch. Once it is over, it is simply admitting defeat to smoke a cigarette from relief.

The coffee break cigarette

Breaking the habit

1 Avoid smokers at your coffee break time.

2 Go to a non-smoking area.

3 If it is the tea and coffee that makes you want a cigarette, change your drink as suggested for breakfast time to a cold drink, to soup, to fruit juice or to an alternative hot drink like Oxo, Bovril, or chocolate. If none of

Fighting temptation

1 Go and talk to a non-smoker.

2 If you find that your fingers are itching because you miss the feel and the handling of a cigarette, occupy your fingers by doing the crossword puzzle, or the Rubic cube during your coffee break. Or if you are a woman, bring knitting or crocheting to work.

3 Distract yourself by reading a

these are available, don't drink at all. Have an apple or an orange.

paper or a book or if you have a portable stereo, listen to some music on your headphones.

The telephone cigarette

Breaking the habit

1 Move your telephone to another part of the room. Just put it on another side of the desk, so that you have to use the opposite hand from usual.

2 Place your cigarettes well out of reach. Never carry your lighter or matches on you.

3 Make sure there are no ash trays near the telephone.

4 Keep a pen and paper next to all the phones so that you can doodle while talking, to occupy your spare hand.

Fighting temptation

1 Make a simple rule that you will not smoke while on the telephone.

2 Pick up a piece of paper or a document, especially if it is relevant to the phone call so that you don't have a free hand.

3 If the telephone cord will allow, walk up and down while taking the telephone call instead of sitting down.

The before and after-work cigarette

Breaking the habit

1 Change your routine completely when you get to work. For instance walk up the stairs instead of using the lift. Hang your coat in a different place. Arrange your desk in a different way. Have a few encouraging words with a non-smoker. Start the day by making a list of everything you have to do instead of having a cigarette.

2 Change your routine at the end of the day in exactly the same way.

3 Instead of ending the day by smoking think about the evening ahead, the meal that you are going to eat, the things that you have to do before you get home, on the way home, what you will do when

Fighting temptation

1 Don't be tempted any more to have a drink with your friends when the work is over before going home.

2 Distract yourself by doing something quite interesting after you have finished work. You might go shopping or drop in at the travel agent and plan your next holiday, take the brochures home, visit a hobby shop or see a non-smoking friend.

you arrive at home (no you won't have a cigarette).

The working cigarette

Breaking the habit

1 Remove cigarettes, matches, lighters, ash trays from the desk.

2 Remove cigarettes, ash trays, lighters, etc. from the room in which you work.

3 If your kind of work permits, change your working routine. You could make a rule that you won't smoke if your hands are dirty. You might re-arrange your office so that you work in a different part of the room or get a different perspective of the room.

Fighting temptation

1 When you want a cigarette, don't sit down; walk up and down the room, or go into another part of the building and chat to a colleague or go and see your secretary.

2 Keep something on your desk or in your pocket that will occupy your fingers like worry beads, or a pad and a pencil so that you can doodle or a pile of paper clips or a simple magnetic toy. If the place where you work has a window, it is not a bad idea to just wander over to the window and concentrate on what is happening outside, just let your mind turn to something different.

The cigarette at the end of the day

Breaking the habit

1. If you unwind when you get home with a drink you may find that for a week or so you are just not going to have to drink either. Remember that the money you save on not smoking will enable you to buy better quality drink when you have got to the stage of drinking without needing a cigarette.

2 Change your getting home routine completely. Sit in a different chair. Take the dog for a walk. Go and see what the children are doing. Go and see if you can help your partner. If you have a hobby, go straight to it and take it up where you left it off.

Fighting temptation

1 Distract yourself with some kind of activity as soon as you get home. There are always some odd jobs to be done around the house. Make a list and start working through them.

2 Take up a new hobby and make it a resolution that you spend half an hour or an hour doing it as soon as you get home.

3 Start eating at a slightly different time. Bring supper forward so
that you can go for a walk after it
or go for a walk before supper.

The cigarette after dinner

Breaking the habit

1 If you usually have a cigarette
sitting at the table with a cup of
coffee, don't stay at the table, have
your coffee in another room.

2 If you find a cigarette an essential accompaniment to the after-
dinner tea or coffee, stop drinking
it and substitute another hot or
cold drink.

Fighting temptation

1 Go for a walk after supper or
make it a special time for an activity that will really distract you.

2 Make a list of all the projects
that you want to tackle within the
next few months, and start tack-
ling them.

3 Phone a non-smoking friend
and plan an outing.

The evening cigarette

Breaking the habit

1 Change your evening routine
completely, enrol at night classes
so that you have to spend some
evenings away from home. Take
up a new hobby that you do as a
group, or a sport or a sports club.

2 Give some time each evening to
your partner or your children.
Decide that every evening you are
going to watch television together,
go swimming together, play games
together.

Fighting temptation

1 Distract yourself with anything
that you find really absorbing.

2 Go for a walk.

3 Get out of the house. Go to the
cinema. Visit a friend. Go to the
Theatre. Join a local club.

The cigarette before going to sleep

Breaking the habit

1 Change your bedtime routine
completely including bath time,
brushing your teeth, your night
clothes, making a late drink,
watching television, reading in
bed. Anything that breaks the
habit.

2 If you usually have your last

Fighting temptation

1 Distract yourself by going over
the events of the day. Don't get
worked up or resentful about
something that has happened.
Concentrate on your achievements.

2 Plan tomorrow, make a list if
you like.

cigarette in bed, stay up and read or watch television until you are ready to fall asleep.

3 If you usually have your last cigarette before going to bed, go to bed a few minutes early and read instead.

3 Think about your success of going without cigarettes during the rest of the day and there is only a minute or so to go before you can notch up another day without cigarettes.

The middle of the night cigarette

Breaking the habit

1 Don't keep cigarettes by the bed or in the bedroom.

2 Keep a drink of fresh fruit juice or a piece of fruit by the bed in case you wake up.

Fighting temptation

1 Have a newspaper or book by the bed to distract you if you wake and can't sleep.

2 Keep a radio by the bed so that you can listen to music or a portable stereo with headphones. You might find that you become so relaxed that you go to sleep with the headphones still on.

3 If your mind is really churning keep a pad and pencil by the bed so that you can list things that you are going to do next day to sort out your problems.

The inner resources – How to use them

All of us have more will-power than we think. You may never have tapped the strength and resources you have. One of the ways we can find our own inner strength is to manage *stress* and control it. Research has shown that the best way to do this is learning how to relax. Once you know that you can cope with stressful situations and you have learned how to relax, most anxieties and problems seem smaller and more manageable and you will also have gained self confidence in your ability to cope. Part of this self confidence will be because you have discovered the ability of how to cope without cigarettes.

Controlling stress

All of us are stressed and nobody can escape the effects of stress. A colleague, Dr John Farquhar from Stanford University in California, has studied the way stress can effect the body and has also devised some very successful ways of controlling it. Before you can control stress, however, you have to know what your particular stressful situations are and how stress effects you. One of the ways you can do this is to keep a log book for a few days of the things that stress you, how much they stress you and the effect they have on you. Anything that makes you feel tense or anxious should go down in your log book.

Here are three samples that John Farquhar and his colleagues would consider typical.

date ....

Stress or tensions felt	Time of day	Where? Doing what? With whom?	Thoughts or feelings	Response to stress
Tight stomach	7.30 am	Getting ready for work	Worried about being late	Hurried more
Headache Tight neck muscles Tiredness	2.30 pm	At work tried to straighten out a serious problem	Frustration	Got angry with secretary and colleagues
Heart racing Tense muscles Tight grip on the steering wheel as I drove home	6.15 pm	In the car on the way home from work in a traffic jam	Very angry	Made several unsuccessful attempts to pass slow cars

If you are the sort of person who reacts badly to stress, and most smokers do, you will gain insight into how much discomfort is caused by stress when you make an inventory of your behaviour under stress. This betrays your tension and anxiety alike, and examples are given here. Why don't you circle the number in the box that reflects how often you are under stress.

Behaviour	Often	A few times a week	Rarely
I feel tense, anxious or have nervous indigestion	2	1	0
People at work and/or at home make me feel tense	2	1	0
I eat and/or drink and/or smoke in response to tension	2	1	0

I have tension or migraine headaches or pain in the neck and shoulders or insomnia	2	1	0
I have difficulty in turning off my thoughts at night or at weekends for long enough to feel relaxed the next day	2	1	0
I find it difficulty to concentrate on what I am doing because I am worrying about other things	2	1	0
I take tranquillizers or other drugs to help me to relax	2	1	0
I have difficulty finding enough time to relax	2	1	0
Once I find the time it is hard for me to relax	2	1	0
My work day is made up of many deadlines	2	1	0

maximum score 20   my score ....

Anyone with a score of between fourteen and twenty has a tension level which is greatly above average and is probably very stressed. A score between ten and thirteen means that you are certainly stressed more than average and you are feeling the tension. A score of six to nine is about average and anything below that means that your life really is not very stressful.

You now know how much stress you have to cope with, but you can also take an inventory of what you do under stress. This will be useful in handling anxious moments. Again you can score yourself in the table that follows to find out how you react to stress:

Behaviour	Never	Seldom (Once or twice a week)	Often (Practically every day)	Very frequently (At least once a day)
Hurriedness - eat and/or move fast	0	1	2	3

Talking - speak fast in an explosive manner. Unnecessary repetitions interrupts others	0	1	2	3
Listening - must have things repeated because of innattentivenes	0	1	2	3
Worries - express worries about small things or things that you can do nothing about	0	1	2	3
Anger and hostility - get angry at yourself and at others	0	1	2	3
Impatience - try to hurry others and become frustrated with your own pace	0	1	2	3

maximum score 18   your score ....

Answering these simple questions should give you an understanding not just of the kind of stress in your life but the way it is produced and the way you react to it. You now know yourself rather well, and you should have pinpointed some important barriers that you have to get over and some attitudes and beliefs that you have to change along with some of your habits, even if they are well entrenched.

Stress management plan
This will help you with your own action plan for change. Stopping smoking is breaking a deep rooted habit and may mean significant changes to your life-style. This plan can help you to do it. To do it you have to make an effort, because you are going to have to learn to acquire two basic skills which may be quite new and foreign to you. These skills are *deep muscle relaxation* and *mental relaxation*. Once you have mastered these techniques, you will not just be able to deal with stress and give up smoking, you will be able to deal with almost any of the problems that life throws at you.

Deep muscle relaxation
This is a technique that was devised at the Stanford Heart Disease Prevention Centre. Don't expect to learn it immediately. It may take a little time, but it is time and effort well spent. Not only does it help you to cope with stress, but it also helps to lower your blood pressure, and decreases the chances of your getting headaches. It

will help you sleep better and feel less anxious. Here is the drill:

1 Find a quiet place and lie on your back in a comfortable position, or if this isn't possible sit comfortably, then close your eyes.

2 The next part of the drill involves your right hand if you are right-handed or your left hand if you are left-handed. Begin by tensing your right hand for just a moment, and relaxing it by letting it go loose. Actually tell your hand to feel heavy and warm. Moving up the right side of your body to the forearm, your upper arm, the shoulder, the foot, the lower leg and the upper leg, go right round the right side of your body. Then do exactly the same thing with the left side of your body. Your hands, arms and legs should feel heavy, relaxed and warm. Give yourself a few seconds for these feelings to develop.

3 Next try relaxing the muscles of your hips, and let the relaxation flow up from your abdomen into the chest. Don't try to tense these muscles, just tell them to feel heavy and warm. You will find that your breathing starts to slow down, and wait for this to happen.

4 Now let the relaxation go up into your shoulders, your jaw and the muscles of your face, with special attention to the muscles around your eyes and in the forehead. Get rid of any frowns. Finish up the drill by telling your forehead to feel cool.

You should practise this drill twice a day if you can, for fifteen to twenty minutes each time. Even a few minutes, as little as three, is better than nothing. The best time to practise is just before meals and an hour or later after meals. Once you have mastered the technique of deep muscle relaxation, you are ready to go on to mental relaxation.

Mental relaxation
Mental relaxation really means clearing your mind of any stressful thoughts, anxieties and worries, and you can do this through the following drill:

1 Just let any thoughts flow through your head. Freely associate.

2 If any thought recurs, stop it by saying 'no' under your breath.

3 With your eyes closed, imagine any calm scene. The most calming is probably a clear blue sky and a calm blue sea, or an object that has no detail. Do try to see the colour blue, because this has been found to be a particularly relaxing colour.

4 Think very hard about your breathing and become aware that it

63

is slow and natural. Concentrate hard on your breathing, and follow each breath as you inhale and exhale.

5 By now you should be feeling calm and rested. You may find it helpful to repeat a soothing word such as love or peace or calm, or a word with less symbolism such as breath, earth, laugh. Think of the word or even a calming sound like 'ah' silently in your mind when you are breathing outwards.

6 Remind yourself to keep the muscles of your face eyes and forehead relaxed and tell your forehead to feel cool.

When you have mastered the mental relaxation drill, deep muscle relaxation and mental relaxation drills should be done together. They are fairly easy to combine once you have mastered them. You should practise the combination of deep muscle relaxation and mental relaxation drill twice a day. Until you have mastered your skills, you should practise them frequently. It may take a few weeks for you to master them completely, and achieve the well-being that comes from relaxation and managing stress.

There are two other things that you can do to help your body to cope with stress. These are instant relaxation and imagery training. Once you are successful at deep muscle relaxation and mental relaxation you should be able to achieve partial deep muscle relaxation and partial mental relaxation within thirty seconds. This is the way to practise instant relaxation:

1 'Arrange' your body comfortably. The best way is to sit comfortably. You can also teach yourself to stand comfortably, even when you are waiting in a queue or just before a stressful experience.

2 Take in a deep breath and hold it for five seconds. Count to five slowly. Then breath out.

3 Tell all your muscles to relax.

4 Repeat this two or three times until you are completely relaxed.

5 Imagine as pleasant a thought as circumstances permit, such as I am learning how to relax, or imagine a pleasant scene. Peaceful countryside or a beautiful view, or a sunset.

Imagery training helps you to use your imagination by breaking down your mental blocks to get more in touch with your body so that you can control it. Sometimes it is quite difficult to learn, but here is a simple test. Think of your left hand and make it feel warm. Then imagine your right thigh and make it feel warm; make it feel heavy. Now try two harder tests. Imagine that one leg is heavier than the other. It may seem odd at first but it is worth practising to get control of the feelings in your body through your imagination. Once you can do these tests easily, you will find deep muscle relaxation simple and that won't be the only benefit. You should be able to control your body to keep away headaches, migraine attacks, lower your blood pressure, and cope with pain.

Incidentally, you are well on the way to being able to cope with stopping smoking. You will be able to handle the most difficult cigarettes of the day, the greatest cravings and the worst temptations. You will be able to overcome the sense of failure, if like some people, you succumb to temptation or just absent-mindedly have the odd cigarette. You won't throw the sponge in. You will increase your dream of being a non-smoker and become even more determined to kick the habit.

Anticipating the commonest worry – weight gain

Many people who are contemplating giving up smoking, think of weight gain as the inevitable outcome, and even use it as an excuse not to give up smoking. Very few people who stop smoking put on more than a few pounds, and just as many people keep their weight steady or even lose some weight – you needn't put on any at all if you prepare yourself properly.

The statistics show that the average weight gained by people giving up smoking is about three pounds, and that is nearly always lost again very quickly. There is no reason to be concerned or worried about gaining weight. You can use exactly the same relaxation methods and exercise (see page 62) to handle weight problems. Remember relaxation and exercise suppress the appetite, decrease the desire for sweet foods and are therefore very helpful in controlling weight. There is no doubt that giving up smoking improves the sense of taste, and you may find that your appetite increases. But there is absolutely no increase in the desire for sweet things. The reason why most people put on weight is that they succumb to the desire to nibble in place of smoking and eat snacks of foods that are high in calories and low in nutrition such as sweets, chocolates, cakes, biscuits and sugary drinks. This is usually because they are easily available. If low calorie snacks were readily available then you would eat them with as much enjoyment in the place of high calorie foods. You have to prepare for this eventuality. Make sure you don't have high calorie nibbles like potato crisps, salted peanuts, biscuits, sweets and chocolates in the house. Instead have a stock of low calorie nibbles (see page 66).

If you are in any doubt, it is much more important to give up smoking than to worry about your weight or even to put on weight. It is better to put on a few pounds and give up smoking than not to give up smoking. Anyone who has the resolve and determination to give up smoking can easily shed the few pounds they have put on while doing it. So if you feel you can't deal with controlling your weight and giving up smoking at the same time, forget it. Leave the weight, and deal with one thing at a time. Give up smoking.

Some people do deal with both things at once in the following way:

1 You can go on a diet and lose a few pounds in the weeks before you decide to stop smoking. This way you may have up to half a stone to play with in case you put on weight.

2 Start eating a balanced diet. This is one which is:

– low on empty-calorie foods, such as sweets, chocolates, cakes, biscuits, fried foods, jam, rich sauces etc.

– low on fats of all kinds, both animal fats, including dairy products like full cream milk and cheese and vegetable fats as well.

– high in roughage such as root and green stringy vegetables, whole grains like brown rice and things made with wholemeal flour, bran, cereals.

– low on animal protein, there is no need to eat meat more than three times a week, red meat once a week, substitute fish or poultry.

– low on any processed or highly refined foods and high on natural, fresh and uncooked foods.

3 Stock up on low calorie nibbles such as:

– any fresh fruit, any raw vegetable, low fat *plain* yoghurt, cottage cheese, the hard low fat cheeses, such as those from Switzerland.

– keep a kitchen jar with sticks of celery and sticks of raw carrot.

– low calorie drinks.

– low calorie diebetic sweets if you have to chew, or sugarless gum.

– skimmed milk, it has fewer calories than unskimmed milk.

– try an artificial sweetener instead of sugar in your tea and coffee.

– low calorie soups for drinks; low calorie salad-dressing.

The average man who isn't engaged in heavy physical work needs three to three and a half thousand calories, and the average woman around two thousand calories a day. If you feel inclined, you can buy a calorie counting book of all the common foods at any book-shop, tot up your calories for the day and make sure you stay within your allowance. Within a few days you know the calorie value of every food you eat and it becomes second nature.

Preparing your environment

This really falls into a few main categories:

1 Prepare the *people* you know. You have got to have the help and support of your *family*, so make sure that everyone is on your side and they have very good warning of when you are going to stop. Make sure they know the exact day when you are going to stop so that they can help make it easy for you and be a source of constant encouragement.

You also have to prepare your *friends*, who can make or break your efforts if you have an active social life. Tell them what you want from them and ask them to give you all the help they can.

You have also got to make sure that the *people at work* are going to help you. Find at least one person where you work who is a non-smoker or who has given up smoking, and ask them if you can call on them or speak to them at any time when you are in difficulties or if you are tempted or if the craving seems too great to control, but ask everyone around you at work to help you.

2 You have got to prepare the *places* where you spend your time. So you have to prepare your *house*. If your partner is a non-smoker it is easy. If your partner smokes you have got to ask for co-operation. If you possibly can you should get rid of all traces of cigarettes and cigarette smoking out of the house, no cigarettes, no ash trays, no matches, no lighters. If your partner smokes ask if the ash trays can be limited in number. They could be covered or confined to one or two rooms. After all if you are sharing a house, part of it should accommodate your desire to be a non-smoker. There is no reason why all of it should be contaminated with cigarette smoke and signs of smoking.

You have got to make exactly the same preparations *at work*. It is well nigh impossible to dictate that people don't smoke in certain places at work except the canteen, but you can ask people not to light up cigarettes when they are near you, and you can warn them that you will move away if they do. If necessary ask if you can be in a part of the works where fewer people smoke.

3 And now the crunch – prepare the *time*: the last part of your preparation to stop smoking is to choose your own special day some time next week – and STOP. Good luck!

6 Hard Facts III

How you are harming your heart

At any age there are more deaths among smokers than non-smokers. Of those people who die earlier than they should because of smoking, heart disease claims 31%, other diseases of the arteries including strokes claim 21%, lung cancer claims 19% chronic bronchitis and emphysema claim 10%, and the remaining 19% are caused by other smoking related conditions. The number of deaths due to coronary heart disease has been rising steadily over the last forty to fifty years and is now the leading cause of death in many developed countries. In Great Britain over 30,000 men and over 10,000 women between the ages of thirty-five and sixty-four die from coronary heart disease, and more than 10,000 of these deaths are directly attributed to smoking. Under the age of sixty-five, smokers are about twice as likely to die of coronary heart disease as non-smokers, and heavy smokers about 3½ times as likely. The chances of having a heart attack are four times more likely in heavy smokers than non-smokers, and two to three times more likely in moderately heavy smokers.

About a quarter of all people who are affected by coronary heart disease are symptomless and appear to be quite well until they suddenly have a heart attack; only about one in three of those who die survive long enough to be seen by a doctor. You don't have to be old to be at risk – cigarette smoking is associated with an especially high risk of sudden death in younger men who smoke cigarettes.

In most cases therefore, prevention is the only hope, and based on avoiding likely causes, the importance of avoiding smoking cannot be over-emphasised. In the face of such risks, it is difficult to know how a smoker can continue to smoke, knowing that the risks of a heart attack fall dramatically after a smoker quits. Most of the studies that have been done, show that the extra risk of heart attack due to smoking is cut in half within a year after stopping. Theoretically speaking, if all the excess risk of heart disease in smokers could be abolished, there would be about 10,000 fewer deaths each year from coronary heart disease in men and women of working age in Great Britain.

There are several ways in which smoking and nicotine may increase the risk of heart disease. Many medical studies have shown that angina, which is heart pain brought on by effort, is associated with cigarette smoking. In some people, smoking can bring on angina even when they are at rest. Furthermore, smokers find that they can walk shorter distances after smoking a cigarette because of the angina pain. The effect is not so marked with low nicotine cigarettes, but it is still there, even with cigarettes that contain no nicotine at all, so angina may be due to the amount of carbon monoxide there is in the blood of smokers which stops the heart muscle getting as much oxygen as it needs.

The level of carbon monoxide in the blood has been shown to be the best indication of which people are at risk from a heart attack. In a very large study carried out on workers in Denmark, it was found that people with more than 5% carbon monoxide levels in their blood had a twenty times greater risk of developing disease of the arteries, including coronary heart disease.

Nicotine and carbon monoxide work together to encourage the development of coronary heart disease. Both produce two effects on the heart which make it more likely for a smoker to have a heart attack. Carbon monoxide reduces the oxygen carrying power of the blood and it may also help the passage of cholesterol through the walls of the arteries so narrowing them down. Nicotine increases the work done by the heart. It also makes the heart muscle more irritable, and this may lead to irregularities of the heart beat. Nicotine also encourages thrombosis.

There is no doubt that some people are at special risk due to a *combination* of various factors, the most common ones being raised blood cholesterol levels, high blood pressure and cigarette smoking. If you don't take any exercise, if you are subjected to a lot of stress which you can't handle, if there is a family history of diabetes, if you suffer from diabetes, and if you are a woman and take the contraceptive pill, then your risk factors are increased. There is a certain sort of personality which is more liable to suffer from coronary heart disease. This is the so-called type 'A' personality. You are an 'A' if you are competitive, impatient and striving.

Coronary heart disease is uncommon in people who have only one risk factor. Research has shown that the most important single risk factor is raised blood cholesterol level, which is becoming more and more common in industrial countries where there is an excessive diet of rich food, particularly saturated and animal fats. In countries where cigarette smoking and high blood pressure are common, coronary heart disease is rare when the average cholesterol level of the population is low.

Where two or more factors occur together, the danger increases, so it is possible to identify people for whom smoking is a particular hazard. The risk of combined factors can be worked out by simply multiplying separate risks. However, in a recent study carried out in Britain it was found that whatever the severity of any other major risk factor, fatal heart attacks were higher in cigarette smokers than in non-smokers. The highest risk of smoking was in men who also had high blood pressure and high blood cholesterol. This can be seen in the following picture.

Smokers are more likely to die of Heart Disease

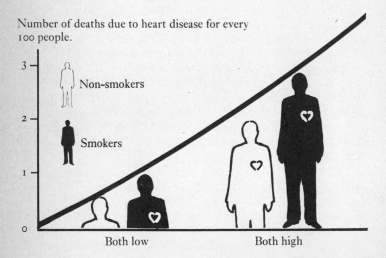

Number of deaths due to heart disease for every 100 people.

The easiest way to reduce your risk is of course to stop smoking, but using this information medical examination and laboratory testing can pin-point those people for whom smoking is particularly dangerous. It should also make smokers seek medical advice if they want to find out for themselves just how important it is for them to give up smoking.

There is another disease of the arteries which is even more closely associated with cigarette smoking than coronary heart disease. This is hardening of the arteries of the leg and of the main trunk artery leading from the heart which supplies all the other blood vessels in the body. Over 95% of patients who have disease in the arteries of the leg are smokers. This disease causes pains in the legs (called intermittent claudication) to the extent that sufferers may not to be able to walk 100 yards. The risk is particularly great in diabetics.

If people are discovered to have this condition and continue to smoke, they are likely to develop gangrene of the legs and possibly to need subsequent amputation. Cigarette smokers are also more likely to suffer from strokes than non-smokers. Death from bursting of the aorta is six times higher in cigarette smokers and ten times higher in those smoking 25 or more cigarettes a day.

Several surveys have shown that there is hardly any increased risk of coronary heart disease in people who smoke pipes and cigars. This is because they are usually light smokers, and rarely inhale the smoke. Contrary to what you would expect there is hardly any reduction in the risk of coronary heart disease in smokers who change from cigarettes to cigars or pipes. This is because such smokers smoke to inhale, and they continue to inhale cigar or tobacco smoke, and therefore keep the level of carbon monoxide in the blood as high as it was when they were smoking cigarettes.

If a cigar or a pipe smoker inhales the smoke they run just as high a risk of dying from coronary heart disease, lung cancer, bronchitis, emphysema and other smoking related diseases as do cigarette smokers.

The continuing story of Mr Petherbridge

Mr Petherbridge is now 40 years old. He says he is smoking 30 cigarettes a day but quite often this creeps up to 35 and occasionally is nearer 40. He has a cough most of the year round, and it is not confined to the morning. Bronchitis each winter is taken for granted. Over the last few years he has been wheezing and he has needed to take medicine to open up the air passages.

He had to give up sports years ago. If he has to run for any length of time he not only gets out of breath but he has pain in the chest. He notices that his chest pain is brought on earlier if he tries to run after smoking heavily. His doctor has told him about the statistics on chronic bronchitis, lung cancer and heart disease, but Mr Petherbridge continues to smoke. He feels for a man of 40 that his disabilities are not very great. In any case he hasn't heard of many smokers who have died of lung cancer or a sudden heart attack. He feels those kind of things happen to other people.

Lung cancer is a killer, but it isn't anywhere near as frequent a killer as coronary heart disease. What is more, it doesn't strike as suddenly, and at 40 Mr Petherbridge is a statistic in a group of male smokers who are likely to die suddenly from heart disease. Because he smokes more than 25 cigarettes a day, he is in the highest risk group.

The death-rate increases with the number of cigarettes you smoke

Deaths in a year for every 100,000 men

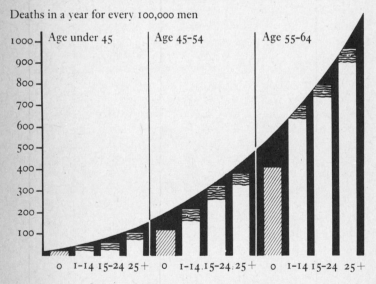

Cigarettes smoked daily

At his age, Mr Petherbridge is running 15 times the risk of dying from a heart attack compared to someone who doesn't smoke. If he only reduced his cigarettes by ten a day, he could lower his risk to 9 times and if he could smoke under 15 cigarettes a day, the risk would be only about 6 times as great. The picture shows that as Mr Petherbridge gets older, his risk of dying compared with non-smokers gets less, but the number of deaths associated with smoking still increases. So for the next five years, Mr Petherbridge is running the highest extra risk over a non-smoker that he will ever run of dying prematurely from a heart attack due to his smoking. If he can survive the next five years, his risk of a heart attack will continue to get worse, though his extra risk over that of a non-smoker will become slightly less.

It is possible to see how Mr Petherbridge could affect his life expectancy now at the age of 40 if he stopped smoking. A vast number of studies have been carried out throughout the world to examine all the effects of smoking on health, and also very importantly to see how health, mortality and life expectancy could be affected by stopping smoking. This picture shows the results of just one.

From the moment you stop smoking your risk of dying from Heart Disease drops

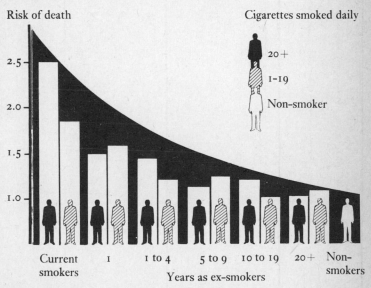

The graph gives you some idea of how much Mr Petherbridge could have done for himself if he had given up smoking. It shows the death rates among men who stopped smoking compared with other men of the same ages. The men were classified as non-smokers, light smokers (1–19 cigarettes a day) and heavy smokers (20 or more cigarettes a day). The picture shows that both light and heavy smokers have a steadily declining risk of dying after stopping smoking. Even though he had smoked as many as 35 cigarettes a day, Mr Petherbridge could have put himself into this statistical group of men who stood an increasingly good chance of *not* dying if he had given up smoking.

At 40, Mr Petherbridge is suffering from angina but he has not yet had a heart attack. What if he does? What are his chances of having another heart attack, possibly fatal, if he continues to smoke, and would his chances be lowered if he stopped smoking? Take a look at this picture.

Continuing to smoke after a Heart Attack increases your chance of having another

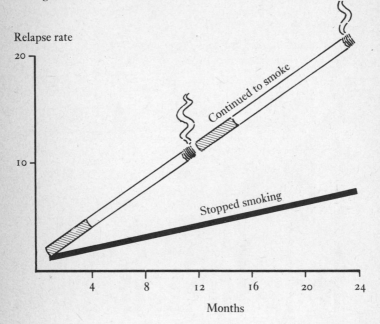

This picture shows quite plainly that there are nearly double the number of subsequent heart attacks in continuing smokers compared to those who stopped. If you are someone who has had a heart attack, and is still smoking, this knowledge should make you stop NOW.

You may wonder about the health warning that appears on most packets of cigarettes and in advertisements for cigarettes that 'Most doctors don't smoke'. Here are the results of their stopping.

Doctors are having fewer Heart Attacks, other men are having more

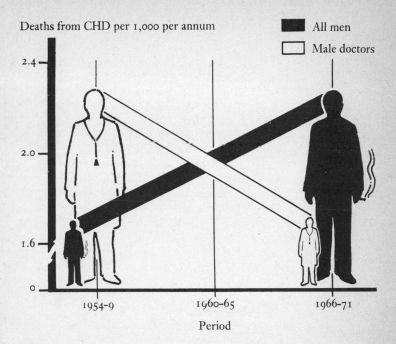

Deaths from CHD per 1,000 per annum

■ All men
□ Male doctors

2.4

2.0

1.6

0

1954-9   1960-65   1966-71

Period

This picture shows how the death rate from coronary heart disease in doctors changed between 1954 and 1971. All these doctors were under 65 years of age. Before 1954, doctors were dying at a faster rate than other men, but since 1954, when doctors read about the association of smoking and serious diseases, their death rate has consistently fallen. Compared to doctors, the death rate for other men has consistently risen, so that in 1971, the positions have been reversed. This reversal is entirely due to doctors giving up smoking and the trend in all other men for smoking to increase.

7 Stopping

This chapter is about actually stopping smoking – the day you stop, and the first few days that follow. I will describe some of the things you may be feeling, some of the difficulties that you will have to cope with. Many people find it a lot easier than they ever thought it would be. But whether you find it is difficult or easy, you have achieved something very great. You have changed your attitudes, you have changed your behaviour and you have broken a habit.

If you find it quite a struggle, take heart. Most people discover that it doesn't last long, so give it a chance. Take one day at a time. Remember, each day without a cigarette is a success.

Nearly everyone says that they can give up smoking for a couple of days, and many people boast that they have done. Like Mark Twain you may have done it thousands of times. The majority of people in this predicament worry about whether they are going to have the strength of will to continue. Very often you worry because you may be suffering withdrawal symptoms. People who have smoked heavily, and have always inhaled deeply are suddenly without the nicotine which they used as a stimulant when they were tired and as a tranquillizer to calm them down when they were tense and anxious. Research however has shown that these feelings rarely last more than a few days, and if you can keep going through the first three or four days, you are definitely over the worst. It will never be as bad again.

The feeling of wanting another cigarette – the craving – nearly always comes on in bouts, spasms that reach a climax. Here are a few of the things that you can do when the craving gets really strong:

1 Remember that the craving will pass within a few minutes, and all you have to do is to get through that short time.

2 Distract yourself with anything: any kind of activity, any change of scene, any change of mood. Switch on the television

set, start reading a book, take up a job that needs finishing. Try and find something that really requires your concentration.

3 Drink a glass of cold water. This seems simple, but it is an excellent remedy, and your mouth actually feels as though cigarette smoke will taste repellent.

4 Take any kind of exercise – walk round the garden, take the dog for a walk, suggest you go for a walk with your partner, play a game of football out in the garden or in the street. Activity helps you get over the craving.

5 Try to keep your hands occupied. Worry beads can be good enough. Why not a Rubic Cube? Take a pencil and paper and jot down some of the jobs that you have to do or make a plan for tomorrow. Write a letter to a friend.

6 Boost your morale by telling yourself that years of smoking are holding you hostage to the desire to smoke, and it is bound to be hard to break a habit of several years. But why should you be hostage to such an unhealthy habit?

7 Remind yourself that you have to *learn* to stop smoking just as you learned to start smoking, and like many other things in life, the learning process can be difficult and requires some effort. You are going to make that effort. You have made quite a substantial investment already in giving up smoking. Don't waste that investment now. Don't weaken.

8 The first few times the craving comes, it may be difficult for you to handle, but very soon you learn how to cope with those difficult moments according to what suits you best. Don't expect to be good at it at first. Every time you conquer it you are learning a little more about yourself, and you are becoming better able to overcome the craving next time it happens. Don't forget it will happen less and less often, and every time you will find it easier to overcome.

9 Try to talk to someone who is a non-smoker or someone who has given up smoking, a neighbour or friend, or just get hold of someone on the telephone who will sympathise with you and talk you through your bad moments. There really ought to be a Smokers' Anonymous.

10 One of the best things that you can do if you are tempted to have a cigarette is the following routine:

STOP!

Close your eyes.

Take one deep breath very slowly.

Count to five.

Breath out very slowly.

Take nine more deep breaths slowly as described.

This routine is very similar to you inhaling a cigarette deeply and you will find the sensation very pleasant even perhaps mimicking the way you used to smoke. The other advantage of doing this is that it is extremely calming and helps you to relax. By the time you have completed it the craving has had time to disappear.

11 Remind yourself that nearly nine million people in Great Britain have given up smoking. Many of them have gone through exactly the same difficulties as you are going through, and they have managed to stop. You can do it too.

12 Whenever you are coming up to a moment that you have nailed down as one of the most difficult cigarettes of the day, take the '*breaking the habit*' or '*fighting temptation*' action that you have decided on and planned to do well ahead of stopping.

13 Re-read pages 54–59 to remind yourself which of these '*breaking the habit*' or '*fighting temptation*' actions you have decided to take. It will help your will-power just to re-read them.

14 When the craving gets really bad, go over your stress control and relaxation techniques that you have been practising since reading Chapter 5 – pages 62–65 – to remind yourself, re-read them.

15 During the first few days there is no harm in spoiling yourself in some way. Don't hesitate to give yourself small treats and small rewards at the end of every successful day or just after conquering one particular time when the craving was really bad.

The day you stop smoking should be really special. You should have taken quite a lot of care in choosing which day you will stop. You should have made it easier on yourself. If you are someone who finds that you smoke a great deal at work, then it's making it extra hard to try to give up during the week. You should choose Saturday or Sunday. On the other hand if you are someone who smokes to relax and you do most of that at the weekend, then it's just silly not to take advantage of doing it mid-week when you smoke fewer cigarettes.

If you can, mark out the day with some kind of special routine or activity. Make it a special day by changing your routine completely. If you have children, and what you would really like is a day on your own to please yourself, get your partner, a friend or a relative to take the children off your hands for that day. Start off with a leisurely routine that you don't normally have time for, a lazy, luxurious bath for instance. Then put on your favourite clothes. Go out and do some shopping, meet some friends for lunch, have your hair done, even a facial. Arrange in the afternoon to go to the theatre or an exhibition, and then later have a night out. Celebrate the fact that you are stopping and mark it out as quite different from all other days. If you are thoroughly enjoying yourself (as long as you make sure that all your friends know that you are stopping smoking, don't offer you cigarettes, don't smoke while they are with you and give you every possible encouragement) you should find the first day much easier to get through.

If you want, you can make the day before you stop special too, by clearing all the ash trays out of the house (as long as your partner agrees), getting rid of every sign of cigarettes such as matches or lighters. You could even make an occasion of smoking your last cigarette as though it were a funeral ceremony, then throwing the rest of the cigarettes away, burying the past and starting on a new, healthier phase of your life.

Nearly everyone will notice within the first few days that their appetite is coming back. This is your body getting back to normal and behaving normally. It's not something that you should avoid or try to bring under control. It is something that you should enjoy. What you should do however, is to make sure that you are eating the right kind of food, and you should have made preparations according to your plan as outlined in Chapter 5 to have the right kind of foods available so that when the urge to eat comes, nutritious low calorie foods that you *like* are readily available. One of the reasons why people tend to put on weight is that they eat the first foods which are available, and more often than not these are fattening foods like sweets, cakes and biscuits. Make sure that there are very few of these kinds of foods around in the house, but lots of other kinds of nibbles as outlined on page 66. So enjoy your new found appetite and use it wisely.

Also start to enjoy the new sensation of food tasting better. You will discover all sorts of flavours and nuances in food which had been masked or even obliterated by the taste of tobacco in your mouth. Eat your food slowly and enjoy every tasty mouthful.

This will help you feel satisfied on quite a little food, and will help to avoid putting on weight.

Coping with the craving

Some research done at Stanford University shows that the following way is excellent for helping you to cope with the craving to have a cigarette. Unlike some of the tips that I have given you before, it doesn't involve distracting yourself but actually *facing* the craving and examining it. It has proved very successful for other smokers, so it may be worth your trying it. It's just another weapon you have in overcoming your own war with cigarettes. This technique helps you to *suppress* the urge to smoke.

How to suppress your urge to smoke

1 When the craving comes, concentrate hard on it. Put everything out of your mind except the craving.

2 Now, slowly step by step go through what happens as you inhale the smoke: you are breathing in the suffocating fumes from a fire; the air is hot and irritating, it makes your tongue hurt and your eyes sting; it's scratching at the glistening lining of your throat and air passages; its corrosive chemicals bite into your delicate tissue and reach every crevice; the smoke bathes the soft pink tender air spaces, drenching them in tar; the air cannot get into the spaces, the oxygen can't get into the blood, the smoke gets there first; you exhale stale air; your breath smells unpleasant; your partner turns his or her head away as they catch a whiff of your halitosis.

3 Concentrate hard on all these unpleasant images as hard as you can until you really feel them. If they get into your consciousness you should rapidly become pretty disgusted with yourself and the craving should wane.

4 Your urge to smoke will be abolished if you go on seeing negative images and so now you can reward yourself. Start with relaxing and go through your relaxation drills (see page 62–65). By the time you're relaxed, the urge will have gone.

5 Now, think pleasant thoughts starting off with the benefits of not smoking. Think of something peaceful. Think of a future treat or date you're looking forward to. Imagine what a good time you're going to have. Start thinking of some way to reward yourself NOW. It need only be small and sometimes, self-esteem is

enough. Feel how relaxed and energetic you are.

6 Have your reward. *NOT a bar of chocolate.*

What to do if you are encouraged to have a cigarette

Even though you may have warned everyone around you someone may inadvertently offer you a cigarette. You may be one of those people who finds it quite easy to refuse and feels extremely proud to say 'No thanks I don't smoke'. On the other hand it may catch you at a weak moment, and you may have to struggle rather hard not to accept it. Here are some of the things that you can do – they have been tried and tested by a team of behavioural scientists at Stanford were smoking cessation was part of a heart health programme.

What to do if you're encouraged to have a cigarette

The kind of arguments you may face	*How to overcome them*
1 You're so irritable for Heaven's sake have a cigarette.	1 That's because my body is still getting used to doing without nicotine. A cigarette would do no good. I'll get rid of my jumpiness with some exercise.
2 You'll probably put on weight. It's well known, smoking keeps your weight down.	2 No I won't, I've planned what I eat. I eat a bit more but I exercise more, and that keeps the urges to *eat* and *smoke* under control.
3 You've been smoking for ages, wouldn't you rather just keep on?	3 Never, I feel very proud to have quit after so long and I'm fitter than I've ever been.
4 Come on, how can just one cigarette hurt?	4 Yes it would. I've put in a lot of hard work to kick the habit, and I wouldn't undo it for anything.
5 You'd be keeping me company if you had a cigarette.	5 *You'd* be keeping *me* company if you stopped smoking.
6 Why not have this very low tar, low nicotine cigarette, it	6 Yes it will, I could find myself going straight back on

can't hurt you?

to my old brand, and anyway carbon monoxide in the blood is worse for heart attacks and strokes than tar and nicotine. I'm not satisfied with half measures, I'm a true NON-SMOKER.

7 Why not have a cigarette – you're going to die sooner or later.

7 No, I'd rather die later than sooner, and by the way smoking may speed up the ageing process.

If you do have a cigarette

No matter how hard you are trying, you may give in to the temptation to take a cigarette, or you may absent-mindedly take a cigarette, because the habit of smoking is so ingrained. When a stressful moment occurs, you may subconsciously or automatically just reach for a cigarette and only realise what you're doing when you're half way through smoking it. *This is not a moment to lose heart and throw in the towel.* Many people have done this and go on with doubled resolution and are successful in giving up smoking completely. What you should try to do instead is to learn from your experience.

Examine why you had the cigarette. Were you unprepared? Were you taken off your guard? Had you become complacent? Was it a particularly bad moment of stress, and you had forgotten how to control it and how to relax? (Remind yourself by reading page 62–65). Could it have been a situation that you might have avoided, or could you have used your fighting off technique? (See page 54). Were you very tired, irritable, frustrated, psychologically at a low ebb? Decide how you are going to cope with these moments in the future. Re-read chapter 5.

Rest assured this is a temporary lapse in your will-power. You are undoubtedly strong enough to give up smoking and your will-power will return. Keep telling yourself that you are going to succeed, and you will succeed and go straight back to your programme of stopping as though you haven't taken a cigarette. And most important of all just because you have taken a cigarette, *you are not a failure.* Repeat this to yourself over and over.

To maximise the possibility of your success during the first few days of stopping smoking, beware of the two arch villains – over-confidence and complacency. Statistically speaking, you are only a non-smoker when you have gone without cigarettes for a year. Undoubtedly the first week is the hardest. If you can get through that you are 90% a non-smoker, so enjoy your success, but never relax your guard.

A lot of very good things will start happening within a short time of you stopping smoking. We have already mentioned a few such as the return of a healthy appetite, and food starting to taste better. You will probably get the feeling that your health is increasing daily. This is not imagination, it really is. Every part of your body is recovering from the deleterious effects of smoking, but particularly your lungs. You will find you are breathing more easily within two or three days, that you are less out of breath when taking any kind of exercise, even walking upstairs, or running for a bus. You will find that if you are playing a sport you can play for longer without getting puffed. You will find that your heart doesn't thud the way it used to when you run.

For most smokers, the smokers' cough will have disappeared by the end of the first week. Others may notice that it gets worse for a few days before it gets better. This is because the lungs are getting back to normal, and are starting up their natural cleansing action with a vengeance. They are cleaning out the poisons and excess mucus which have been collecting in the lungs for years. The 'muck and rubbish' is being cleared out of the lungs by the newly-returned sweeping action of the cilia (see page 43). Once your lungs are thoroughly cleaned out, your smokers' cough will go completely. However, if it does not go away, you should visit your doctor.

Added to all this you will find that your breath smells sweeter, nicotine stains have gone from your fingers, your body, hair and clothes smell sweeter, the acrid smell of cigarette smoke has disappeared from the house. There are no messy dirty ash trays to look at or clean up, and you are saving money – put it in the 'Quit Kitty', and save it up for a treat.

Here are a few more of the benefits that you will be enjoying within a few days of giving up smoking. On the face of it they don't seem very great, but until you have given up and experienced them, you don't know just how much they are going to mean to you.

1 You have a feeling of pride in yourself, and pride in your strength of will, pride in your achievements, a feeling of greater self confidence, a feeling of having conquered something that is really quite difficult to do.

2 You will have the praise of the others around you, particularly your children if you have any. I remember one of the best moments, indeed one of the greatest rewards that I had as the result of giving up smoking, was hearing one of my sons boasting about the fact that his mum didn't smoke any more.

3 You have joined an élite. You have joined a group of people who are unquestionably more sensible than the people who continue to smoke. You have responded to logic and good reason. *You have joined the non-smokers.*

4 You may get quite a thrill – I did – to start hearing yourself say 'No thanks I don't smoke'.

5 Your efforts to stop smoking may have cost you quite a lot, but you have bought a healthier life and a longer life, possibly by as much as ten years.

6 You have automatically put yourself in a lower risk category for developing lung cancer, heart disease, chronic bronchitis, emphysema, peptic ulcer, cancer of the panchreas, and several other smoking related diseases.

Giving up smoking for some people may be quite hard. For a very few it may be one of the hardest things they have ever had to do. Console yourself with the truism that many people die as the result of smoking, but nobody has ever died from giving up smoking.

8 Hard Facts IV

In this chapter I am going to discuss some special aspects of smoking, which include:

1 Smoking and women
2 Smoking and pregnancy
3 Smoking in public places
4 Cigarettes and the media
5 Smoking Advertising

Smoking and women

More women are smoking than ever before. Men seem to have responded to anti-smoking campaigns during the last ten to fifteen years better than women, so that the proportion of men who smoked in 1961 was 60% whereas it was less than 50% in 1975. The proportion of women who smoke has stayed at around 40% during that time. There are two main reasons why this has happened. Firstly, smoking is still seen as a mark of independence in a woman, so many have not got to the point of taking anti-smoking publicity seriously.

It is not just that the number of women who smoke now is greater, it is also the number of cigarettes they smoke. Up until the 1940's it was considered not quite the thing for a woman to smoke. By 1950 the average woman in Great Britain was smoking about half as many cigarettes as a man, but now the women have made up much of the difference, girls are starting to smoke earlier than they ever did, and in some western countries, there is a greater proportion of young girls smoking than young boys. It is the first time that this has ever occurred in the history of smoking. In 1979, more American teenage girls were smoking than boys. Out of every ten teenage girls, nearly four are smoking 20 cigarettes a day.

It would seem that the western way of life helps a man to

become a non-smoker whereas exactly the same factors hinder a woman. The profile of the successful male ex-smoker is that he is married, a college graduate and has three or four children. He probably smoked for less than ten years before giving up. His wife probably disapproves of him smoking, and will support him in his efforts to stop. All these factors seem to have the opposite effect in women. For a woman, marriage and parenthood means that she is less likely to have stopped smoking. A disapproving husband or the presence of children make it harder instead of easier to stop.

While generally, there seem to be more smokers in the lower socio-economic classes, this is not so for women. In a survey done among men and women managers, it was found that 42% of women managers smoked, compared with only 37% of men. Women find it harder to stop smoking than men. They have lower success rates in all socio-economic classes, every kind of professional occupation and all age groups. Even when groups are highly motivated, men are twice as successful at stopping smoking than women, irrespective of the method they use. Another sad statistic is that women who give up smoking seem to return to cigarettes more rapidly than men. A Canadian study showed that after a year, one-third of the men were true non-smokers whereas only one-fifth of the women had been successful.

This adherence to smoking shows up in the health statistics. In 1977 8,500 British women were killed by lung cancer, giving Britain the third highest female lung cancer death rate in the world. It has been worked out that one woman dies of lung cancer every hour of every day throughout the whole year, almost all because of their smoking.

Cigarettes are a major cause of heart disease in women, just as they are in men, and it is the number one killer of women just as it is in men. 65,000 women in England and Wales died of heart disease in 1979. This means that more women die of heart disease than all forms of cancer combined together. Irrespective of other risk factors, a woman who smokes twenty cigarettes a day is twice as likely to die of a heart attack as a woman who doesn't smoke at all. A woman who smokes and takes the oral contraceptive pill as well, will multiply the risk of dying of a heart attack caused by smoking.

Thus, a woman who smokes 25 cigarettes a day, and takes the oral contraceptive pill is about 40 times as likely to have a heart attack than a woman who neither smokes nor takes the pill.

The other two main diseases caused largely by smoking, chronic bronchitis and emphysema kill as many British women as everybody who is killed in road accidents.

Women smoke for all the same reasons and in all the same situations as men. And then there are a few added pressures. Women who are working in a predominantly male environment, particularly if they are in supervisory or managerial positions have been shown to be under greater stress than men. Women who are tied to the home with small children get more bored than men. Both of these reasons *drive* women to cigarettes. Smoking is also associated with 'liberation'. For decades, smoking was disapproved of in women. It is only comparatively recently, say the last 30 years, that it has been accepted. Many women began to smoke and kept on smoking because they associated cigarettes with an image of worldliness, ambition and success. Women also smoke because they believe that it will keep them thin. While they are smoking they are not eating and so smoking is often used mistakenly as a slimming aid. And finally there are the pressures through the media, films and advertising that encourage women to smoke (see page 90).

Smoking and pregnancy

A woman should give up smoking for herself. That reason, added to the desire to have a healthy child, demands that she gives up smoking during pregnancy.

There is no question that smoking during pregnancy has a harmful effect on the baby. Mortality rates are higher and the birth rate is lower in babies of mothers who smoke. Women who smoke have babies who, on average, are about half a pound lighter than mothers who don't smoke. In other words each cigarette a woman smokes during pregnancy decreases the weight of her baby.

The incidence of prematurity, (a baby born less than 5½ lbs in weight) is almost double the rate in smokers compared to non-smokers. The effect of smoking is greatest in the second half of pregnancy. It has been found that women who cut down on their cigarettes or stop smoking before the twentieth week of pregnancy tend to have babies of similar birth weight to women who don't smoke.

It is not really known why smoking retards the growth of a human baby, but there are three possibilities.

1 The chemicals that are absorbed from cigarette smoke directly

affect the growth of the baby detrimentally.

2 Mothers who smoke may eat less than non-smoking mothers, and therefore the baby doesn't get the same nourishment, and therefore cannot grow properly.

3 Nicotine may reduce the blood supply of the placenta, and therefore interfere with the nourishment of the baby.

It is conceivable that nicotine absorbed from cigarette smoke can have a direct effect on the developing tissues of the baby, by causing narrowing of the blood vessels of the placenta. In addition to this, whatever the level of carbon-monoxide in the mother's blood, it becomes more concentrated in the baby's blood, and thus lowers the amount of oxygen which the blood can carry. Research has shown that the more carbon-monoxide in the baby's blood the smaller its weight is at birth.

Spontaneous abortion is more common among smoking mothers than non-smoking mothers, and there are more still-births than deaths in the first week of life. Mothers who continue to smoke after the fourth month of pregnancy are increasing the risk of their baby dying within the first week of life by nearly a third over mothers who don't smoke. The death rate in babies rises with the number of cigarettes smoked, up to about ten a day. After that it makes very little difference. A mother can't afford to smoke even a few cigarettes.

It is particularly important for a mother who is 'high-risk' not to smoke because this will increase the possibility of something going wrong. So, for instance if a mother has suffered a still-birth in the past, it is absolutely crucial that she doesn't smoke the next time she is pregnant because this could greatly increase her chances of having another still-birth.

The effect of a mother smoking while she is carrying her baby shows well after the baby is born. Some research has shown that at the age of eleven, children of smoking mothers are half an inch smaller and three months behind in their reading age than children of mothers who didn't smoke. They also appear to be clumsier and less good at copying drawings.

The babies of smoking parents are at great risk during the first year of life when they have a tendency to develop bronchitis and pneumonia. Even if only one parent smokes, children are more susceptible to chest infections than the children of parents who don't smoke. It has been suggested that the household air contaminated by cigarette smoke could directly damage a child's developing lungs.

Smoking in public places

Many non-smokers object on purely aesthetic grounds to breathing air which is polluted by cigarette smoke. In addition to this there are very good health grounds for objecting. People who breathe in air contaminated with cigarette smoke are 'passively' smoking, and there are dangers inherent in this. This is particularly so in small enclosed places, such as a taxi, a car, a bus, a railway compartment and an office where there are several heavy smokers. It has been shown that a non-smoker may inhale as much smoke in one hour as an average cigarette smoker inhales from one cigarette. If a non-smoker is continually exposed to air laden with cigarette smoke, his or her health will be damaged and they will be running the same risks as a smoker who smokes five cigarettes a day.

Recent evidence from Japan has suggested that the non-smoking wives of smokers may suffer a higher risk of lung cancer than the wives of non-smokers. But this association is still questioned. There is no doubt however, that people suffering from asthma, allergies or chest complaints are uncomfortable in smoky rooms and at the very least non-smokers find smoky atmospheres unpleasant.

Smokers should probably have the right to smoke, but equally non-smokers should have the right to a smoke-free environment in cinemas, theatres, restaurants, work and most importantly, in hospital.

The restriction of smoking in public places is important in at least two respects. First of all it counteracts the impression that smoking is a normal acceptable, social convention. It also protects the non-smoker from a smoky environment. Possibly the most important effect is that it gives the newly stopped ex-smoker protection against relapse.

At least 60% of all people in Great Britain are non-smokers, and a recent survey showed that most of these people and even 50% of smokers would like to see restrictions on smoking in shops, restaurants, cinemas, planes, coaches and buses. What we should be working towards therefore, is an attitude whereby *non-smoking* is usual in public places, and special provisions are made for people who want to smoke.

It is staggering that a better example is not set in hospitals where there are very few restrictions on smoking, where ash-trays are often provided on bedside tables, cigarettes are freely available in the hospital shops, and are even brought around to the wards on trolleys. A public opinion survey has shown that nearly 70% of smokers and nearly 80% of non-smokers would favour a complete ban of smoking on hospital wards. To put it the opposite way round, only one quarter of the people who are admitted to hospital would like to have the freedom to smoke in hospital. It should therefore be the aim of the hospital authorities to make smoking an exception in hospital rather than the rule, so that non-smoking becomes the normal practice.

Cigarettes and the media

It is ironic that Benson and Hedges can claim to be 'purveyors of cigars and cigarettes to Her Majesty the Queen', and yet there is an undoubted link between smoking and the deaths of Edward VII, George V, Edward VIII, and George the VI.

Edward, the Prince of Wales, who set many fashions through-out Europe, was the first to introduce the habit of smoking cigarettes immediately after dinner. Mr Hedges, of Benson and Hedges was asked to provide miniature cigarettes especially for the ladies, and thus the habit began.

The media has always been at great pains to put over the idea of smoking as strong, dashing and romantic in men, e.g. Hum-phrey Bogart, James Cagney, John Wayne, Steve McQueen, and sultry, sexy and sophisticated in women, e.g. Marlene Dietrich, Lauren Bacall, Rita Hayworth. Naturally enough, both men and women, eager to emulate the glamour of film stars, felt they acquired some of the glamour by smoking. Ironically, both Humphrey Bogart and Steve McQueen died from lung cancer. Even today, in films and in the theatre, if a part calls for sophis-tication and worldliness, particularly in a woman, then the char-acter uses cigarettes as a means of projecting this kind of image.

Smoking and advertising

The tobacco companies have a great deal to answer for. The Managing Director of Carreras Rothman stated in 1976, 'The aim, to keep people smoking, has been achieved'.

While tobacco manufacturers claim that their advertisements are aimed at promoting *brands* of cigarettes, and are not intended to encourage smokers to smoke more, they inevitably condone and promote the social acceptability of smoking.

Some smokers even regard cigarette advertisements as show-ing that there can't be any harm in the habit otherwise the gov-ernment wouldn't allow cigarettes to be advertised.

Certain practices of the tobacco manufacturers such as collecting coupons deter a cigarette smoker from stopping.

To counteract criticism, tobacco manufacturers sponsor more and more sporting and artistic activities in an effort to associate smoking with healthy and attractive pursuits. This distracts the public from the true association of smoking with illness, or thinking that smoking is undesirable.

The tobacco manufacturers put forward the argument that if they withdrew sponsorship from sporting and artistic events, then sports would stop and opera would die. This is not so. When Rothman withdrew its sponsorship of the British Hard Court Tennis Championships, Coca Cola took over. The Welsh Rugby Union refused tobacco sponsorship on principle, but continued to exist and indeed thrive showing that tobacco sponsorship was unnecessary for success.

There are examples around the world showing that it is feasible to prohibit the promotion of tobacco in national advertising. Norway in 1975 and Finland in 1977 banned advertising of cigarettes. At the same time part of the revenue from tobacco taxation was set aside annually for health education. There is no reason why the same should not happen in Great Britain.

The continuing story of Mr Petherbridge

Mr Petherbridge is now fifty and is still smoking around thirty-five cigarettes a day despite the fact that he is never without a cough and more often than not spits up yellowish green phlegm. This means that his lungs are chronically infected. The signs show in many ways:

1 He cannot climb a flight of stairs without getting out of breath and has to stop half-way up in order to get his breath back.

2 He cannot now walk any distance at a brisk pace. He can't run at all.

3 The maximum distance he can walk fairly slowly is about two hundred yards when he has to stop to get his breath back.

4 Every winter he has serious attacks of bronchitis which take him to his bed for anything up to six weeks and which require long courses of antibiotics before his chest is clear.

5 For the last four years he has had at least one attack of bronchitis which was so severe that he had to go to hospital and was

put in an oxygen tent. On two of these occasions the bronchitis was complicated by pneumonia.

6 His skin is constantly a greyish-blue colour, particularly around the mouth showing that the blood is not being efficiently oxygenated when it passes through the lungs.

7 Recently he has noticed that his ankles have started to swell because fluid is collecting there. His Doctor has told him that his lung disease is causing a back pressure on the heart and his heart is unable to take the strain. The swelling of his ankles is the first sign that his heart is beginning to fail.

Mr Petherbridge, at fifty, is a statistic: smoking will almost certainly cause him to die of heart failure in less than 10 years, unless he stops.

Each year thirty thousand men and women die from bronchitis and emphysema in the United Kingdom. In the age group thirty-five and over more than twenty thousand men die from the effects of chronic bronchitis directly due to smoking.

Such is the severity of Mr Petherbridge's emphysema that he is destined to be one of that group. Even though these statistics have been pointed out to him he continues to smoke.

It is known that Mr Petherbridge may have inherited his susceptibility to the effects of smoking cigarettes. He belongs to a group of smokers whose lung function has deteriorated very rapidly. There are others in whom the deterioration occurs more slowly. Two of Mr Petherbridge's children, one daughter and one son also smoke and they have already begun to show early signs of developing bronchitis. This means that there may be a deficiency of a certain enzyme which is running through the Petherbridge family and which has passed on through the genes, making them more liable to develop chronic bronchitis and emphysema. This is a development which smoking probably speeds up even though Mr Petherbridge, his son and his daughter are unaware of it.

It takes most cancers fifteen to twenty years to develop. Mr Petherbridge's cancer is already growing in his lung. Its growth is being promoted with every cigarette he smokes. It is spreading microscopically to other parts of his body via his blood. He will die of lung cancer.

9 Staying Stopped

In this chapter I will be looking at some of the things that make it difficult for you to stay stopped, and how you conquer all of them and *stay stopped*.

There is no question that the first week of giving up smoking is the most difficult, but your enthusiasm, your determination and support from your friends may help you to get over this first difficult time. Around about the third or the fourth week things may start to get difficult again. First of all your enthusiasm of the first few days stopping may be wearing thin and your friends and family may no longer be making such a fuss of you. Secondly your will-power may have been worn down because you have had to face lots of difficult moments and your strength of will is being sapped. If you are having a more difficult time than you thought, do please stay with it – it will get easier. It is very important that you keep going through this time. Here are a few things that may help you.

For most people below middle age the pressures to continue smoking are far stronger than the motives to stop and you may as well face up to that. In the following picture, the 'mastery' motive in the list on the left is the wish to show other people that you have the will-power to gain control over the habit. The 'aesthetic' motive describes the feeling that smoking is dirty and messy and the 'example' motive means that you wish to stop, to set a good example to your children and to other people.

The factors that are weighing against these motives to stop are given on the right hand side of the picture on page 94. To be aware of them is to arm yourself to resist them.

To stay stopped, one of the things you have to be convinced of is that the motives on the left hand side of the picture are going to help you more than those on the right hand side. Read them over carefully and think about each one for several minutes from as many aspects as you can.

It is essential that you make a plan to prepare yourself for a

Factors tempting you to restart smoking, and factors helping you to stay stopped

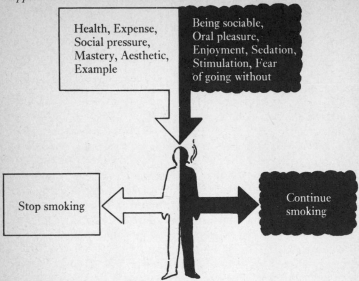

moment of weakness when you may take a cigarette. It should be your own personal plan and you should be ready to put it into operation if the craving becomes great, if you are with smokers or if you are with someone who offers you a cigarette. By now you will have conquered the automatic desire to reach for a cigarette and you should have developed a reflex for putting into action your 'resistance plan'. Here are a few suggestions:

1 Think ahead.

2 Just as you prepared *to stop smoking* now prepare for the stresses of the future.

3 Plan to cope *without* cigarettes.

4 Work out your instant stress control plan (see page 62).

5 Have at the ready your instant relaxation plan (see page 62).

6 Work out well ahead of time what your distraction procedure is going to be, whether it's in a domestic environment, at work or when you're enjoying yourself with friends.

7 If you need to occupy your fingers always carry around something to fiddle with like worry beads or a Rubic Cube.

8 Instead of 'chewing' on a cigarette, chew on something else; always carry around a tube of mints in your pocket and keep chewing-gum handy.

During these difficult weeks, the contract you made with your friend can be of great help. Take it out and look at it, read it through, refer to it when you are feeling weak. Ring your friend up to gain moral support. Talk about the things that you are going to do when you have got to the end of the contract, plan your treat, all these things will help you to keep going through difficult moments.

A few people find that they get depressed several weeks after giving up, but this is quite rare. If you do experience any depression research has shown that you usually get over it quite quickly.

In giving up smoking you are changing your life in a very radical way. The people who get depressed are those that give up smoking without replacing it with something else and that is why it is very important to plan ahead to make sure that you are occupied, distracted and getting help from everyone around you. It certainly does help to find something to do with your hands, especially if it is constructive and rewarding – like doing odd jobs around the house, sewing, knitting, carpentry, car maintenance etc. Try to remember also that you are saving a lot of money, and this will easily pay for any materials that you have to use to keep your hands and mind busy.

If you continue to be depressed go and see your doctor. One of the most important factors in helping people to stay stopped is the support of their family doctor. If you can, try and see your doctor before you stop to warn him or her of your plans. Tell him or her that you will be calling on them to give you support when your will-power weakens. There is hardly a doctor who won't encourage and support you in stopping smoking. Many will do it by example but many more will continue to reinforce your determination by reminding you of the health statistics which show how deleterious smoking is to your health and remind you of all the benefits of stopping smoking.

One doctor in Buckinghamshire has taken his dislike of smoking and desire to help his patients to the point of declaring that he will no longer take patients on to his books who continue to smoke. This is a perfectly rational approach. There is hardly a single organ in the body which is not damaged by the effects of smoking. Any work that a doctor does is diminished by the effects of smoking. This outspoken doctor is saying, 'Why should

I waste my efforts to make you better when you are choosing to make yourself worse?'

During these difficult weeks you will probably wonder if there will ever be a time when you don't want to smoke. Remember someone who has smoked is always vulnerable to starting again, sometimes after a gap of even several years. Don't make the mistake of feeling that it is safe to assume you are completely cured and try just one. An ex-smoker is only one cigarette away from being a smoker. Every time you are tempted try to remember that if you succumb to the temptation you may be back on twenty cigarettes a day within a week. Surely you are not going to waste all this effort?

A lot of people will wonder if various smoking aids work and whether they should try them. Most smoking experts agree and I am with them, that there is no substitute for will-power. Most of them feel that in the first instance you should try to go it alone. Smoking aids should really be reserved for those people who fail initially but still have the determination to give it a second try. By no means all of them work. Here is a brief rundown of the various methods that are available and my opinion as to whether they are valuable.

Hypnosis

We don't know how hypnosis actually works, there is no doubt that it works for some people. Hypnosis can't make you do something that you really don't want to do. Even the most suggestible people are not prepared to act in a certain way if it goes against their nature. For instance it is not possible to seduce someone under hypnosis if they don't want to be seduced. Similarly, it is not possible for someone to give up smoking under hypnosis unless *they really want to do so*. So the criterion for using hypnosis is that you really want to give up smoking in which case you might be helped by it. It is always best to rely on yourself, not on someone else. One of the best parts of giving up smoking is the sense of achievement. You might be denied this inspiration if a hypnotist is taking most of the credit.

Acupuncture

The same remarks can be said about acupuncture. For stopping smoking, acupuncture has a fairly high failure rate, somewhat higher than hypnosis. There is no possibility of it working if, in your heart, you don't really want to give up smoking.

Using Astringents in the Mouth

There are mouth washes, tablets and sprays containing astringents which only taste unpleasant when you start to smoke a cigarette. The taste is absolutely foul, but like all these other aids they *cannot be relied on alone* to help you to give up smoking.

Astringents have to be used alongside one of the plans outlined in Chapter 3. A situation where they may work is when your habit is automatic and you are concerned that you may reach for a cigarette without actually knowing it. If you use an astringent there is no way you can light up a cigarette without noticing it with the very first draw. The effect of an astringent lasts for anything between two and four hours and if you are using them you must continue throughout the day and evening.

Medication

The scientific evidence is equivocal. Some studies have shown that drug treatments to help giving up smoking have been successful and others have found just the opposite. As with everything else it is your approach that is important and the amount of will-power that you have. If you are determined and you have a positive attitude towards giving up smoking they may help.

The active ingredient in most of these medications is lobeline. The manufacturers claim that this substance gives the satisfaction of nicotine without any of the harmful effects. So it really acts as a nicotine substitute. There is no knowing whether it will act for you or not. It is included here, not because it has a high success rate, but so that you are aware of the options open to you.

Nicotine chewing gum

In specialised smoking cessation clinics, there has been quite a good success rate using nicotine chewing gum. You can get it from your doctor but you have to pay for it, it is not available on the National Health Service.

This kind of chewing gum releases nicotine as you chew. It is absorbed through the mouth, gets into the blood stream and affects the brain and the other organs as outlined on page 16, in the same way as nicotine from a cigarette.

Nicotine reaches the blood stream from the chewing gum in the mouth more slowly than from cigarette smoke and it is not as easy to control, so there are special ways to chew it. Your doctor can instruct you and there are instructions on the pack. It takes some practice to learn to control it. One of the dangers of nicotine chewing gum is that people see it as a freely available form of nicotine and find themselves chewing the gum more often than they would smoke. They are taking larger doses of nicotine through the gums than they ever did through cigarettes. While it is, in no way, a 'magic cure', it does supply nicotine while the habits of smoking are being broken.

In the context of specialised clinics where people are reviewed frequently and given enthusiastic support by the doctors, nicotine chewing gum does help people to give up smoking. It also helps a smoker to cut down on cigarettes. However, the successful ex-smoker then has to go through the experience of doing without the nicotine chewing gum. They have to weather the difficult phases of stopping smoking and stopping chewing. It may take several weeks and sometimes even months to give up the gum. On the other hand chewing gum does not have the harmful effects on the lungs that smoking does and therefore it is less important how long it takes to give up the gum.

Some research has shown that chewing ordinary gum can almost be as helpful as chewing the kind that contains nicotine and as yet trials of the nicotine chewing gum have not shown if it has the same success rate in the general population as it does in people who are kept highly motivated by regular attendance at clinics.

Attending a Smoking Cessation Clinic

This is one of the best ways of giving up smoking and if there is a clinic in your area or a self-help group go along and join it.

In this country there are between fifty and a hundred smokers' clinics run by the National Health Service, usually attached to hospitals, to help you to give up smoking. The clinics set out with the aims of this book and do very much the same things as this book is trying to do. They give people information about the health risks of smoking and advice on how to give up. They try to reinforce your determination by showing films and by getting people to talk about their feelings and experiences as they have tried to give up smoking. There are also lectures by successful ex-smokers so that you are constantly reminded that it is possible to give up smoking and often it's easier than you ever thought.

As with everything else a clinic cannot *make* you give up. You still have to make all the decisions and you still have to find the will-power. All that a clinic does is to make it easier for you and to show you in very clear terms that it is worth doing. A useful aspect of a clinic is that you will meet other like-minded people who are interested in doing the same thing as you. This kind of therapy is extremely supportive to people who are trying to change their attitudes, behaviour and way of life in whatever they are doing.

Herbal Cigarettes

Undoubtedly herbal cigarettes are less damaging to your health than ordinary cigarettes but they do still contain some tars and carbon monoxide in the cigarette smoke. They are useful to people who still need to handle a cigarette and want to feel a cigarette in their mouths and also to inhale one. They are less harmful than ordinary cigarettes because they are not at all addictive. There is very little risk of you becoming hooked on a herbal cigarette because they contain no nicotine.

While it doesn't get my wholehearted support because your aim is to give up smoking for good, making the switch from ordinary cigarettes to herbal cigarettes is a substantial step forward. If you find that you can get by on herbal cigarettes for three or four weeks you may as well not be smoking at all because it is extremely easy to give them up. One of the inherent dangers that I see in herbal cigarettes is that people who smoke them very often revert back to nicotine – containing cigarettes. If this happens to you, you really have to bite the bullet and do it properly.

You won't get any satisfaction from herbal cigarettes so there is no point in inhaling them. Stop inhaling immediately. One of the ways you may try using them is as a substitute for the most difficult cigarettes of the day. You can phase them out completely after a week or so. It also gives you an excuse when offered a cigarette to say: 'No thanks I smoke my own brand'. You don't have to give away that you are smoking herbal cigarettes.

Your weight

Even though gaining weight is not the inevitable consequence of giving up smoking, you're still going to have to be vigilant about not putting on weight, so be prepared and follow the plans suggested on page 66. Research among women has shown that one-third of women who give up smoking don't gain any weight at all and some actually lose weight.

Some women, however, do gain a few pounds. You really do have to plan your diet sensibly because your appetite will increase, your food will taste better, your food will be more efficiently absorbed when you stop smoking because smoking actually inhibits the absorption of essential nutrients and this is one of the reasons why smokers are less healthy than non-smokers but also because smoking encourages food to be burned up fairly rapidly.

The main thing is to eat a well balanced diet which is low in empty calories. This way you will remain healthy and you won't put on weight. Another way of looking at it is to decide whether a few pounds, by that I mean two or three, is a bad thing for you. You may have become obsessive about staying thin and this is particularly so in the case of women. If you gain more than seven pounds then you definitely should take steps about it. Ask yourself a few questions and perhaps you may decide that you will just readjust yourself to the idea of being a few pounds over-weight. For instance:

1 Will your life change if you gain a few pounds?

2 Are you really obsessed about being thin?

3 Are you trying to please other people, especially a media image, by trying to stay thin?

4 Which is more important, staying healthy or trying to please others by being as thin as they think you ought to be?

5 Will a few pounds really make you *fat*?

6 Are you a less worthy person for being a few pounds over-weight?

7 Are you valuing your physical appearance more than the health of your body?

8 Is it just a lack of self confidence because you feel you don't have an awful lot to offer other than being slim?

In this way you will release yourself from the straightjacket you may have been living in for years – the glossy magazines' asser-tion that slimness is an essential part of twentieth century living. Your health is far more important. Recent research in America has shown that you will probably live longer if you are a few pounds overweight than if you are a few pounds underweight and the actuarial lists of the ideal weights for heights are actually increasing the ideal weight for both sexes at any given height.

Always be on your guard to staying stopped, remember you are not a non-smoker until you have stopped for a year. Don't fall prey to excuses for one more cigarette such as 'I can always stop again tomorrow'. As soon as you have taken your first cigarette you are a smoker again.

10 Hard facts V

This chapter is the pay off. It outlines what you, as a successful stopper, will have achieved in terms of:

1 generally improved health.

2 a lower risk of lung disease, such as chronic bronchitis and emphysema.

3 a lower risk of developing cancer of the lung.

4 a decreased chance of having a heart attack at any age, and a sudden heart attack which may be fatal if you are young or middle-aged.

5 a decreased risk of developing diseases of the blood vessels.

It will also examine 'what if?' What if you lapse? What if you go back to smoking? What if you think you have failed? This chapter will help to give you a positive attitude towards your lapse so that you won't consider yourself a total failure. It will help you to recover your previous determination and self-esteem and not allow you to go back to your old smoking habits. It will catch them long before they take hold again. I will outline a programme which has been used successfully by people who have relapsed so that you may eventually achieve your goal of being a non-smoker.

So let's take stock. What have you gained by giving up smoking? The list is almost endless, and all of it's good, better than you think. Because you have given up smoking your extra risk of dying before your time disappears in ten to fifteen years. In a long term study of British doctors, twice as many smokers as non-smokers aged 35 or over died before reaching 65. From the moment you gave up smoking you started to cut that risk. You are exactly the same as a non-smoker in anything from ten years onwards.

From the mid fifties to the late sixties deaths fell in the general population by only 7% whereas amongst doctors who stopped smoking, deaths under the age of 65 fell by 21%. You have joined the doctors.

In the case of lung cancer, giving up smoking markedly reduces the chance of dying, so that after ten years the risk is almost identical to that of a lifelong non-smoker. Again evidence comes from the long term study on British male doctors. Among the group of doctors who were smokers, and gave up the habit, deaths from lung cancer have declined. The death rate from lung cancer continued to increase in the general population whereas the death rate from lung cancer in doctors as a whole has fallen dramatically, because most of the smokers among them have stopped.

It also takes about ten years after giving up smoking to reduce the risk of heart disease to approximately the same as that of a non-smoker though the risk starts to go down immediatly you stop smoking. Smokers who stop smoking after a coronary heart-attack are less likely to have another attack than smokers who continue their habit. A study which was carried out in Sweden has shown that stopping smoking halves two separate risks: the number of fatal and non-fatal heart attacks. The risk of a stroke is also reduced. It has been estimated that the lives of between nine thousand and ten thousand people in Great Britain would be saved every year if it were possible to abolish the excess risk of heart disease due to smoking. And this is just the figure for men and women who are of working age. By reference to the same British study in doctors, we know that there's a rising death rate from heart disease in men under 65, whereas the death rate has been falling steadily in doctors of the same age, simply as a result of having stopped smoking.

There's quite a lot of evidence which shows improved functioning of the lungs and lower death rates from bronchitis in ex-smokers compared with people who continue to smoke. There's no doubt that damage to the lungs can be halted by stopping smoking. Several studies of lung function in working men over several years, looking at smokers and non-smokers, have shown that stopping smoking slows down the rate of deterioration even when the damage to the lungs is considerable.

By doing tests of lung function it's possible to identify the smokers who, with only mild abnormalities, will deteriorate to the point of being severely disabled if they continue to smoke. Smokers who run the greatest risk of developing bronchitis and emphysema can be pin-pointed and 'saved'.

One of the excuses that smokers use for continuing to smoke is that there don't seem to be many people around who die as a result of smoking. It's true that only a small number of smokers die in the prime of life as the result of an illness caused by smoking. However the total number of casualties is enormous. Only 16% of non-smoking men will die between the ages of 35 and 64, whereas 28% of men who smoke 15 to 24 cigarettes a day will die, and 36% will die if they smoke more than 25 cigarettes a day. If these proportions are applied to the millions of smokers in Great Britain today, they add up to a shocking number of premature deaths.

The balance between the benefits and harm from smoking is well accepted so it's surprising that large and powerful institutions don't do more to discourage the habit. Trade Unions, for instance, spend time and money in preventing, curing and gaining compensation for industrial diseases. By comparison they have shown little interest in the effects of smoking even though there is infinitely greater harm done by the effects of smoking on the health of trade union members compared to the harm inflicted by industrial diseases. However, that is gradually changing.

The Government could provide a powerful counter-attack on the strength of tobacco advertising by replacing the current ineffective warnings on cigarette packets. Instead of SMOKING CAN SERIOUSLY DAMAGE YOUR HEALTH, there should be the firm and convincing warning which accompanies the tar and nicotine tables published by the DHSS: CIGARETTES CAUSE LUNG CANCER, BRONCHITIS AND HEART DISEASE.

The Health Service could do a great deal more to encourage people to stop smoking, especially if there were a programme for detecting people with a high risk of developing certain smoking-related diseases. It's thought that smokers with fairly minor abnormalities of lung function may be prone to developing severe bronchitis and emphysema. People with high blood pressure and high blood cholesterol may have an increased risk of coronary heart disease. There is even indication of which smokers may be at high risk for developing lung cancer. The DHSS could encourage and support research into methods of persuading these high risk people to give up smoking. If such a project was used to compare the effect of abstinence with a control group who did not stop smoking, we could obtain proof of the relationship between smoking and disease of the heart and lungs.

The majority of people are unaware of how many people suffer impaired health and die prematurely because they smoke cigarettes. Statistics show that deaths due to smoking are at least seven times greater than deaths from road accidents. The death rate from road accidents has been reduced because large sums of money have been spent on advertising campaigns to encourage people to drive more carefully and to make roads safer. The amount of money and effort invested in trying to prevent deaths from smoking compared to this is miniscule.

We are doing very much less in the UK than in other countries. Eleven countries have put a ban on all tobacco advertising. Norway, Finland and Sweden have set up advisory bodies run by the Central Government on how to take action to curtail smoking. They have instituted warnings on cigarette packs which are much clearer than those in England. In Finland £1 out of every £200 of tobacco revenue is invested in public education on the harmful effects of smoking and the benefits of giving up. In a recent survey on the provisions that are made for non-smokers in public places, Britain came a shameful 17 out of 20 in a list of European countries.

Now that you are a non-smoker, why don't you make it your business to be a bit evangelical about it? Give your support to anyone you know who is trying to give up smoking and make it known that you will enter into a contract with someone who is determined to kick the habit. A little agitation never comes amiss and progress is usually made piecemeal, little by little. If there is no provision made for non-smokers in a public place, ask for it. If you go into a hotel room whose furnishings are impregnated by the cigarette smoke of the previous occupant, ask for your room to be changed, and point out the reason for your request. Encourage meetings to be held with a ban on smoking. Think about the various ways you could give the people who don't smoke the same number of choices as the people who do.

How to handle a relapse

If you do experience a minor relapse, you must not label yourself as a failure. This will only result in your feeling inadequate and having many negative thoughts which decrease your chances of achieving lasting success. The greater the failure you feel, the more attractive the invitation to return to your old habit. But you'll waste everything that you've learned and all the efforts you've made. The most important thing you can do is to return to your non-smoking way of life as quickly as possible, even if you've had several cigarettes. You may be able to avoid self-defeatist thinking by going through these following steps, which will help to convince you that you can be a non-smoker again, quickly.

1 Accept that your return to smoking shows that it is still attractive to you. It is this attractiveness of smoking that has exerted its power over you and made you return to it.

2 Go through exactly the same drill as outlined in the previous chapters.

– Think about the reasons why you smoke.

– Think about the ill-effects of smoking.

– Think about the benefits of stopping smoking.

– Decide to stop smoking.

– Prepare to stop smoking.

– Choose a day and stop.

You must choose a day no further than three days ahead. During those three days, decrease your smoking if you possibly can to only a few cigarettes a day. Prepare yourself again for the difficult cigarettes. Work your way through them as outlined on pages 54–59. Enlist the help of your family and friends and gain their support. Don't be ashamed to admit that you relapsed, but say that you're even more determined that you'll give up this time.

3 It's essential that you go through all these steps in a matter of fact way without any kind of breast-beating. Try to imprint on your mind that smoking is unpleasant for both you and other people. It makes you unattractive. Without it you will be a great deal more attractive both to yourself and to others.

4 Whatever you do don't be discouraged. One of the ways of helping to build up your self esteem and also your determination is to go through the drills that I outlined on pages 80–84 on how to suppress the urge to smoke and the arguments you should use to yourself and to others on how to remain a non-smoker.

5 Consider trying some of the aids to giving up smoking described on pages 96–99.

I believe you can do it. If *you* believe you can do it, you can and will. GOOD LUCK!